D1427009

OXFORD MEDICAL PUBLICATIONS

End of Life Care in Nephrology

Published and forthcoming Oxford Specialist Handbooks

General Oxford Specialist Handbooks
A Resuscitation Room Guide (Banerjee and Hargreaves)

Oxford Specialist Handbooks in End of Life Care
Cardiology: From advanced disease to bereavement (Beattie, Connelly, and Watson eds.)
Nephrology: From advanced disease to bereavement (Brown, Chambers, and Eggeling)

Oxford Specialist Handbooks in Anaesthesia
Cardiac Anaesthesia (Barnard and Martin eds.)
Neuroanaesthesia (Nathanson and Moppett eds.)
Obstetric Anaesthesia (Clyburn, Collis, Harries, and Davies eds.)
Paediatric Anaesthesia (Doyle ed.)

Oxford Specialist Handbooks in Cardiology
Cardiac Catheterization and Coronary Angiography (Mitchell, Leeson, West, and Banning)
Pacemakers and ICDs (Timperley, Leeson, Mitchell, and Betts eds.)
Echocardiography (Leeson, Mitchell, and Becher eds.)
Heart Failure (Gardner, McDonagh, and Walker)
Nuclear Cardiology (Kelion, Loong, and Sabharwal)

Oxford Specialist Handbooks in Neurology
Epilepsy (Alarcon, Nashaf, Cross, and Nightingale)
Parkinson's Disease and Other Movement Disorders (Edwards, Bhatia, and Quinn)

Oxford Specialist Handbooks in Paediatrics
Paediatric Gastroenterology, Hepatology, and Nutrition (Beattie, Dhawan, and Puntis eds.)
Paediatric Nephrology (Rees, Webb, and Brogan)
Paediatric Neurology (Forsyth and Newton eds.)
Paediatric Oncology and Haematology (Bailey and Skinner eds.)
Paediatric Radiology (Johnson, Williams, and Foster)

Oxford Specialist Handbooks in Surgery
Hand Surgery (Warwick)
Neurosurgery (Samandouras)
Otolaryngology and Head and Neck Surgery (Corbridge and Warner)
Plastic and Reconstructive Surgery (Giele and Cassell eds.)
Renal Transplantation (Talbot)
Urology (Reynard, Sullivan, Turner, Feneley, Armenakas, and Mark eds.)
Vascular Surgery (Hands, Murphy, Sharp, and Ray-Chaudhuri)

End of Life Care in Nephrology

From advanced disease to bereavement

Edwina Brown
Consultant Nephrologist
Hammersmith Hospital, London, UK, and
Professor of Renal Medicine,
Imperial College London, UK

E. Joanna Chambers
Consultant in Palliative Medicine
Southmead Hospital, Bristol, UK

Celia Eggeling
Lead for Psychosocial Care
Renal and Transplantation Unit
SW Thames, UK

Series editor

Max Watson
Consultant in Palliative Medicine
Northern Ireland Hospice
Belfast, UK, and
Honorary Consultant
The Princess Alice Hospice
Esher, UK

OXFORD
UNIVERSITY PRESS

OXFORD
UNIVERSITY PRESS

Great Clarendon Street, Oxford OX2 6DP

Oxford University Press is a department of the University of Oxford.
It furthers the University's objective of excellence in research, scholarship,
and education by publishing worldwide in

Oxford New York

Auckland Cape Town Dar es Salaam Hong Kong Karachi
Kuala Lumpur Madrid Melbourne Mexico City Nairobi
New Delhi Shanghai Taipei Toronto

With offices in

Argentina Austria Brazil Chile Czech Republic France Greece
Guatemala Hungary Italy Japan Poland Portugal Singapore
South Korea Switzerland Thailand Turkey Ukraine Vietnam

Oxford is a registered trade mark of Oxford University Press
in the UK and in certain other countries

Published in the United States
by Oxford University Press Inc., New York

© Oxford University Press, 2007

The moral rights of the authors have been asserted
Database right Oxford University Press (maker)

First published 2007

British Library Cataloguing in Publication Data

Data available

Library of Congress Cataloging in Publication Data

Data available

Typeset by Newgen Imaging Systems (P) Ltd., Chennai, India
Printed in Italy
on acid-free paper by
LegoPrint S.p.A.

ISBN 978–0–19–921105–0 (Flexicover: alk.paper)

10 9 8 7 6 5 4 3 2 1

Dedication

To Doctor Catherine Chambers, trainee nephrologist, who lived
life to the full, and by her practice enabled others to do so.

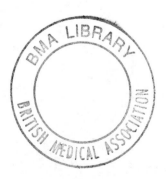

Foreword

This timely collaboration brings together the knowledge, insight, and passion of four experienced practitioners with a deep understanding of their subject. The principles of end of life care have recently been articulated in health policy documents including the National Service Framework for Renal Services and the Gold Standards Framework – in the UK the Quality and Outcomes Framework of the General Medical Services Contract mandated the introduction of registers for chronic kidney disease and palliative and support care from April 2006. Many people with chronic kidney disease should be on both registers. This book provides an invaluable resource for all clinicians caring and prescribing for these individuals.

The honesty is refreshing, advanced kidney disease is not portrayed as asymptomatic – rather the panoply of physical, social, and psychological burdens of living with kidney disease are described and the approaches to their management are discussed. Tellingly the list of potential complications of dialysis is longer than those of chronic kidney disease alone. We are cautioned that clinicians often assume a more favourable prognosis than is justified. At times that avoids the 'difficult conversation' and denies patients 'the truth'. For many patients dialysis is not the bridge to renal transplantation. Dialysis doesn't transform lives – it is often palliative treatment. Given the mortality of dialysis programmes, the authors are right to point out that if the surprise question can't be dismissed immediately in the individual case, conversations should take place and supportive measures should be put in place.

Communication – listening, permitting silence, non-verbal interactions as well as honest conversation are emphasised as the key skills to complement the detailed knowledge base provided here. The importance of family and cultural dimensions in decision–making are highlighted. The nature of the belief systems of the major religions provides a useful insight into the spiritual context of patients and carers.

Helpfully, recent changes in the law and an authoritative account of the General Medical Council guidance provides clear principles in an area that can be frightening and stressful for staff.

A good death is a right we must provide for our patients. This book emboldens the phrase **in conjunction with conventional care for the renal patient** on several occasions. It provides a detailed and joined up approach to palliative and supportive care for the person with kidney disease. It provides the context and identifies the skills which healthcare professionals need – it will benefit patients, carers and staff.

Dr Donal O'Donoghue
National Clinical Director for Kidney Care

Preface

We have written this handbook to try and provide a compact but comprehensive guide to management of patients with renal disease at the end of their life. There is increasing awareness among renal healthcare professionals about the need for good supportive care at the end of life and therefore increasing involvement of palliative care teams. The authors include a renal physician, a palliative care physician, and a renal counsellor. This book has evolved from a previous collaboration in writing (Chambers EJ, Brown EA, Germain M (eds) (2004). *Supportive care for the renal patient.* Oxford University Press) and organizing an annual renal palliative care course.

During our day to day management of dying patients and their families, we have come to realize the need for a practical book that gives basic renal information to the palliative care professional and guides the renal professional through the communication skills and knowledge needed to provide palliative care to their patients. We hope this book will fill this role. It is aimed primarily at doctors and nurses in the renal and palliative care teams, but should be of use and interest to all other healthcare workers involved with the dying patient—pharmacists, dieticians, counsellors, social workers, and psychologists.

The book starts with basic information about the renal patient at the end of life—what they die from and what symptoms to expect and why. It then continues with guidance on controlling pain and non-pain symptoms followed by suggestions to help professionals recognize when the renal patient is dying. Practical ways of enhancing patient, family, and team communication are discussed leading on to a description of supportive and palliative care including how and when it might be accessed. Ethical and legal considerations are discussed before a detailed chapter on end of life care. Spiritual care and care for the carers conclude the book. As a practical guide to management, the book is didactic and represents our own clinical practice. We have therefore used case histories to further illustrate such management in practice. We have left plenty of space for the reader to add their own notes and observations.

We are especially grateful to Wendy Lawson, senior pharmacist at the Hammersmith Hospital, who helped write the drug guidelines throughout and authored Chapter 15, and Ann Banks, renal staff nurse, for giving the nurse's perspective on caring for the dying. We would particularly like to acknowledge our patients and their families who have taught us so much.

Contents

Detailed contents

Contributors

Ann Banks
Carrington Ward
Southmead Hospital
WOT Bristol
BS10 5NB

Wendy Lawson
Department of Pharmacy
Hammersmith Hospital
Du Cane Road
London W12 OHS

Marika Hills
Cancer Services
Somerset House
Southmead Hospital
WOT Bristol
BS10 5NB

Abbreviations

AIDS	acquired immune deficiency syndrome
APD	ambulatory peritoneal dialysis
APKD	adult polycystic kidney disease
ARF	acute renal failure
ASA	acetylsalicylic acid
ASN	American Society of Nephrology
B3G	buprenorphine-3-glucuronide
b.d.	twice a day
BDI	Beck Depression Inventory
BUN	blood urea nitrogen
CAPD	continuous ambulatory peritoneal dialysis
CCPD	continuous cycling peritoneal dialysis
CKD	chronic kidney disease
CMV	cytomegalovirus
CPAP	continuous positive airway pressure
CPR	cardiopulmonary resuscitation
CRF	chronic renal failure
CRN	community renal nurse
CVD	cardiovascular disease
ED	erectile dysfunction
ERA	European Renal Association
ESF	established renal failure
ESRD	end-stage renal disease
ESRF	end-stage renal failure
FSH	follicle-stimulating harmone
GABA	gamma aminobutyric acid
GAS	general adaptation syndrome
GFR	glomerular filtration rate
GHRH	gonadotrophin-releasing hormone
GI	gastrointestinal
GM	glomerulonephritis
h	hour(s)
H3G	hydromorphone-3-glucuronide
HAART	highly active antiretroviral therapy
Hb	haemoglobin
HCG	human chorionic gonadotrophin

HD	haemodialysis
HIV	human immunodeficiency virus
HRQL	health-related quality of life
5-HT$_3$	5-hydroxytryptamine 3
ICD	International Classification of Diseases
IDDM	insulin-dependent diabetes mellitus
IM	intramuscular(ly)
IOM	Institute of Medicine
IV	intravenous(ly)
KDOQI	Kidney Disease Outcomes Quality Initiative
KDOQL	Kidney Disease Outcomes Quality of Life Questionnaire
LH	luteinizing hormone
LVEF	left ventricular ejection fraction
M&M	morbidity and mortality
M3G	morphine-3-glucuronide
M6G	morphine-6-glucuronide
MOAIs	monoamine oxidase inhibitors
NCHSPCS	National Council for Hospice and Specialist Palliative Care Services
NECOSAD	Netherlands Cooperative Study on Adequacy of Dialysis
NHP	Nottingham Health Profile
NHS	[UK] National Health Service
NICE	National Institute for Clinical Excellence
NMDA	N-Methyl-D-asparate
NNH	number needed to harm
NNT	number needed to treat
NPT	nocturnal penile tumescence
NTDS	North Thames Dialysis Study
PD	peritoneal dialysis
pmp	per million population
PMTs	pain measurement tools
po	by mouth (*per os*)
PR	rectally (*per rectum*)
prn	as needed
PTH	parathyroid hormone
PVD	peripheral vascular disease
QALY	quality adjusted life year
q.h.s.	at bedtime
q.o.d.	every other day
q.i.d.	four times a day
RBC	red blood cell
rHuEpo	recombinant human erythropoietin
RLS	restless legs syndrome

RPA	Renal Physicians Association [of the USA]
RPCI	Renal Palliative Care Initiative
RRT	renal replacement theraphy
SC	subcutaneous(ly)
SCr	serum creatinine
SF-36	Medical Outcomes Study Short Form-36
SIP	Sickness Impact Profile
SSRIs	selective serotonin re-uptake inhibitors
STAI	State Trait Anxiety Inventory
stat	immediately
TCA	tricyclic antidepressants
TENS	transcutaneous electric nerve stimulation
t.i.d.	three times a day
UK	United Kingdom
USA	United States of America
USRDS	US Renal Data System
WHO	World Health Organization
WHOQOL	World Health Organization Quality of Life [Assessment]
WNERTA	Western New England Renal and Transplantation Associates

End-stage renal disease

Chronic kidney disease

Chronic kidney disease (CKD) is a major public health problem. As the prevalence of diabetes and obesity increases, and as the population ages, the prevalence of CKD will continue to increase. This is reflected not only in the increasing incidence and prevalence of patients with end-stage renal disease (ESRD) requiring dialysis, but also in the substantial comorbidity found in such patients. Many patients are therefore not going to be suitable for transplantation. Despite the improvements in dialysis care, these patients will experience significant mortality and morbidity and an impaired quality of life.

Definition of CKD

The internationally accepted definition is based on that proposed by the National Kidney Foundation—Kidney Disease Outcomes Quality Initiative (NKF-K/DOQI) workgroup:

- the presence of markers of kidney damage for 3 months, as defined by structural or functional abnormalities of the kidney with or without decreased glomerular filtration rate (GFR), manifest by either pathological abnormalities or other markers of kidney damage, including abnormalities in the composition of blood or urine, or abnormalities in imaging tests; or
- the presence of GFR < 60mL/min/1.73m^2 for 3 months, with or without other signs of kidney damage as described above.

Staging of CKD

- Stage 1 disease is defined by a normal GFR (> 90mL/min/1.73m^2) and persistent albuminuria.
- Stage 2 disease is a GFR between 60 and 89mL/min/1.73m^2 and persistent albuminuria;
- Stage 3 disease is a GFR between 30 and 59mL/min/1.73m^2;
- Stage 4 disease is a GFR between 15 and 29mL/min/1.73m^2;
- Stage 5 disease is a GFR < 15mL/min/1.73m^2 or ESRD.

The majority of patients with stage 5 CKD will require renal replacement therapy (RRT), i.e. dialysis or transplantation. Patients with stage 4 CKD will have many of the complications of renal failure and have a greatly increased mortality risk, particularly from cardiovascular disease. The pharmacokinetics of renally excreted drugs will be markedly affected in both groups, thereby making end of life care difficult.

Prevalence of CKD

Studies in the US and UK suggest similar prevalences for CKD, with approximately 10% of the population having CKD.

- 0.3% population have stage 4 CKD.
- 0.3% population have stage 5 CKD.
- People with hypertension, diabetes, vascular disease, or obesity are at increased risk of having CKD.
- Nhanes studies (general population surveys) in the US show that incidence of CKD stage 1–4 has not substantially changed from years 1988–94 compared to 1999–2000 (8.8 and 9.5%, respectively).

- Prevalence rate for stage 5 CKD (ESRD) has doubled over same time period.
- CKD more common in elderly.
  - Japanese data suggest that over 80% of people aged over 70y have at least stage 3.
  - Median age of starting dialysis in UK is around 65 years.
- There is huge variation in incidence and prevalence of ESRD in different ethnic groups.
  - Incidence of ESRD in South Asian and Afro-Caribbeans in UK is 3–4-fold higher than in general population.
  - In US, compared to Caucasians, the incidence of ESRD in other ethnic groups is also increased: × 4 in American Africans, × 1.5 in Asian Americans, and × 2 in Native Americans.

Causes of renal failure

There are many ways of classifying the causes of renal failure. In the context of this book, i.e. end of life management in renal disease, the majority will have CKD, but some patients will have presented with acute renal failure that has not recovered. As the symptoms of any associated disease have to be managed at end of life, it is useful to list the causes of renal failure with the underlying disease process.

Vascular disease

- People with hypertension, cardiac disease, peripheral vascular disease, cerebrovascular disease (so-called 'arteriopaths') are at greatly increased risk of developing CKD.
- Renal damage due to hypertension, renovascular disease, ischaemic nephropathy.
- Hypertension represents 25% of all primary diagnoses in the USA, but is less frequent (around 9–10%) in Europe.
- Cholesterol emboli.
  - Occur after arteriography or vascular surgery; more rarely spontaneously.
  - Presents as multisystem disorder associated with acute renal failure.
  - Usually renal function does not recover.

Diabetes

- Commonest cause of renal failure in the USA where 44% of new patients starting dialysis in 2001 had diabetes.
- Around 20% patients in UK starting dialysis have diabetes; more common in South Asian ethnic populations than in Caucasian population.
- More common in northern Europe (accounts for around 40% patients starting dialysis in some parts of Germany) than in southern Europe where around 12% of new dialysis patients have diabetes.
- Over 90% will have type 2 diabetes.
- Majority will have vascular comorbidity.

Glomerular disease

- Several types of glomerulonephritis can cause ESRD, but original histological diagnosis does not affect outcome at this stage (unless type that recurs in transplant, e.g. focal glomerulosclerosis).
- More common as a cause of ESRD in younger patients.
- Disease process can be over many years, thereby allowing the vascular complications of hypertension to develop.

Autoimmune disease

- Examples are lupus (SLE), vasculitis, scleroderma.
- Relatively rare cause of renal disease.
- Often multisystem involvement because of nature of disease.
- Patients will often have had treatment with immunosuppression drugs for prolonged periods of time.

- In some patients, disease process is very rapid so they present with acute renal failure that may or may not respond to immunosuppression treatment.

Familial disease
- Most common type is polycystic kidney disease, which is an autosomal dominant condition.
  - Kidneys can be very large resulting in marked abdominal distension.
  - Bleeds into cysts can be very painful.
  - Frequently cysts in liver, which can also be painful.
- Rarer types.
  - Alport's syndrome: hereditary nephritis associated with neural hearing loss and cataracts; variable inheritance.
  - Tuberous sclerosis: autosomal dominant; associated with skin lesions, renal and cerebral tumours, epilepsy, and mental retardation.
  - Von Hippel–Lindau disease: autosomal dominant cystic renal disease associated with a variety of tumours including renal clear cell carcinoma, angioblastomas including retinal angiomas, phaeochromocytoma.
  - Metabolic disorders such as cystinosis, oxalosis, Fabry's disease.

Malignancy
- Renal carcinoma requiring bilateral nephrectomy.
  - At risk of metastases even after removal of original tumours.
  - Renal tumour in only functioning kidney.
- Urinary tract or pelvic tumours causing obstruction.
  - Primary tumours, e.g. prostate, bladder.
  - Secondary tumours causing bilateral ureteric obstruction, e.g. from rectal, cervical, or ovarian carcinomas.
  - Management primarily urological.
  - Dialysis not usually considered for long-term treatment unless patient young and to 'buy' time to allow other treatments time to work.
- Haematological malignancies.
  - Myeloma.
  - Primary amyloid.
  - Presence of renal failure complicates treatment with cytotoxic drugs.
- Complication of nephrotoxic cytotoxic drugs.
- Radiation nephritis.

Infections
- Worldwide, infections are a very important cause of renal disease.
- HIV-related renal disease most common type of renal disease in high risk areas, e.g. sub-Saharan Africa.
- Other infections causing chronic kidney disease are hepatitis C, hepatitis B.
  - These are endemic in some parts of the world.
  - Intravenous drug abusers are at high risk of such infections.

- Acute post-infectious glomerulonephritis, e.g. due to streptococcus.
  - May result in ESRD at first presentation, though uncommonly.
  - Slow deterioration in renal function after initial episode.
- Subacute bacterial endocarditis.
  - Commonly will resolve after treatment with antibiotics, but not always.

Miscellaneous

- Reflux nephropathy.
- Sickle cell disease.
- Analgesic nephropathy.
- Drug-induced:
  - cyclosporin-related renal disease following solid organ transplantation, e.g. heart, lung;
  - Chinese herb nephropathy.
- Secondary amyloid associated with chronic inflammatory conditions, e.g. rheumatoid arthritis, ankylosing spondylitis.
- Toxins, e.g. lead, mercury.
- Congenital and acquired obstructive uropathy.
- Chronic interstitial disease, e.g. due to sarcoid.
- Haemolytic uraemic syndrome.

Transplant rejection

- Chronic rejection is common cause for patients starting dialysis.
- Patients have a disease burden associated with long-term use of immunosuppressive drugs, cardiovascular risk of renal disease.
- May have difficulty with vascular access because of previous dialysis.
- Can be considered for another renal transplant if medically fit, though this may be difficult if high levels of cytotoxic antibodies.

Unknown

- Cause of renal disease is unknown in about a fifth of patients starting on dialysis treatment.
- This is more common in people who present late with advanced kidney failure (stage 4 or 5 CKD).
  - No obvious history of hypertension or proteinuria.
  - Usually kidneys are small on renal ultrasound, so technically difficult to biopsy.
  - If kidneys are biopsied, histology consistent with end-stage kidney disease (sclerosed glomeruli, interstitial fibrosis), but no indication of original cause.

New patients on dialysis

The 2005 UK Renal Registry Report[1] gives the data for patients on renal replacement therapy (RRT) in the UK during 2004. It is compiled from complete data for adults from Northern Ireland, Scotland, and Wales and an extrapolation from the 83% of the English population covered.

- **Acceptance rate.** Just over 6000 adult patients were accepted for RRT in the UK during 2004; this equates to an acceptance rate of 103 per million population (pmp).
  - Acceptance rate is unchanged from 2003.
  - ESRD is more common in men; annual acceptance was 127 pmp for men and 74 pmp for women.
- **Change in incident rate.** Progressive rise in incident rate seen since 1982 seems to have slowed or stopped in the last 2–3 years. This could be due to:
  - improved predialysis care;
  - increasing proportion of patients, particularly older ones, selecting conservative management rather than dialysis.
- **Median age** of patients starting RRT in UK is 65.1 years. Patients starting on dialysis continue to get older.
  - Since 1998, median age of patient starting RRT has increased by 1.5 years in England and by 6.2 years in Wales.
  - Since 1998, percentage of incident patients aged over 75 has risen from 18% to 23% in England and from 20% to 29% in Wales.
- **Diagnosis.** Percentage distributions of primary renal diagnosis by age and gender in patients starting dialysis in 2004 are shown in Table 1.1.
  - Diabetes remains the most common primary renal diagnosis.
  - Incidence of diabetic renal disease higher in centres with greater percentage of non-White patients.
- **Dialysis modality.** 71% patients started on haemodialysis (HD), 26.5% on peritoneal dialysis (PD), and 2.3% with a pre-emptive transplant.
  - This is a major change from 1998 when only 57.7% started on HD.
  - Wide variation between renal units ranging from 42 to 100% of patients being on HD at day 90.
  - HD more frequently first treatment in Wales and Scotland than in England.
  - Age is major factor: 80% patients over age of 65 were on HD at 90 days compared with 64.3% of patients < 65 years old.

Table 1.1 Percentage distribution of primary renal diagnosis by age and gender in 2004[1]

Diagnosis	Percentage of patients			
	<65y	>65y	All	M:F ratio
Aetiology unknown	18.5	27.6	23.0	1.6
Glomerulonephritis	13.3	7.7	10.4	2.4
Pyelonephritis	7.5	6.4	7.0	1.2
Diabetes	21.4	14.7	18.0	1.7
Renovascular disease	2.7	12.2	7.5	2.0
Hypertension	5.7	5.3	5.5	2.1
Polycystic kidney disease	8.0	2.8	5.4	1.0
Other	15.3	12.5	13.9	1.3

Reference

1 UK Renal Registry Report 2005.

Patients on renal replacement therapy

- **Numbers**. Around 38 000 adult patients were on RRT in the UK at the end of 2004 (equates to a population prevalence of 636 pmp). 61% were male. There has been a 5.9% per annum increase in numbers with a 23% overall increase over the 5 years 2000–2004.
- **Age**. In terms of numbers of patients, prevalence of RRT is greatest in age range 55–65 years.
  - Maximal prevalence rate is in age band 65–74 (1460 pmp) overall, but is different in men (80–85 year age band: 2065 pmp) and women (65–74 year age band; 1,073 pmp).
  - Prevalence rates are increasing annually in all age bands over age of 30 with largest increase in 55–85 year bands.
  - Transplant prevalence greatest between ages 40 and 60 years.
  - Dialysis treatment prevalence greatest between ages 60 and 80 years.
- **Primary renal disease**. Percentage distributions of primary renal diagnosis by age and treatment in patients on RRT in 2004 are shown in Table 1.2.
  - Most common diagnosis is glomerulonephritis for age < 65 years (22.3%) and diabetes for age > 65 years (13.4%).
- **Treatment modality**. Overall 44.9% patients are transplanted, 42.1% are on HD, and 13% are on PD.
  - Proportion of prevalent dialysis patients on PD varies from 0% to over 40% at individual UK renal units.
  - As shown in Table 1.3, use of modality depends on age whether patient is diabetic or not.

Table 1.2 Primary renal disease in prevalent RRT patients in 2004 from UK Renal Registry Report 2005[1]

Primary diagnosis	Percentage aged		Percentage having	
	<65y	>65y	Transplant	Dialysis
Unknown	16.4	24.8	39	61
Glomerulonephritis	22.3	13.4	57	43
Pyelonephritis	14.5	9.1	56	44
Diabetes	11.6	13.2	27	73
Polycystic kidneys	9.6	8.1	58	42
Hypertension	5.1	7.4	40	60
Renovascular	1.4	8.7	14	86
Other	15.5	10.3	48	52
Not sent	3.5	5.0	35	65

Table 1.3 Treatment modality related to age and type of diabetes from UK Renal Registry Report 2005[1]

Treatment modality	Percentage of patients with		
	Type 1 diabetes	Type 2 diabetes	Non-diabetic
Patients aged < 65y			
Haemodialysis (%)	38	62	29
Peritoneal dialysis (%)	18	22	11
Transplant (%)	44	16	59
Patients aged > 65y			
Haemodialysis (%)	76	75	63
Peritoneal dialysis (%)	15	18	14
Transplant (%)	8	7	24

Reference

1 UK Renal Registry Report 2005.

Comorbidity

Introduction

Not only is comorbidity a powerful predictor of early and late mortality in patients with ESRD, but also the severity of comorbidities in individual patients will have a powerful effect on their quality of life. Many patients with ESRD, particularly in older age groups, will have one or more comorbidities. These can be divided into:

- cardiovascular disease (cardiac, peripheral, or cerebrovascular) which is much more common in patients with renal failure than in the general population;
- diabetes—as primary diagnosis or coincidental, i.e. not cause of renal disease;
- coincidental disease, e.g. malignancy, chronic lung disease, liver disease, arthritis, etc.

The UK Renal Registry does attempt to collect comorbidities in patients starting on dialysis. As this is time-consuming for individual clinicians, the data collected are incomplete. Thus, in the 2004 report, information on comorbidity is only available in around 40% of the incident patients. These data (Table 2.1) show that two-thirds of patients starting dialysis over the age of 65 years have at least one comorbidity.

Factors affecting comorbidity

- **Age**. Frequency of all comorbidities increases with age, apart from being a smoker.
- **Diabetes**. Higher prevalence of vascular disease amongst diabetic compared with non-diabetic patients.
  - Fewer diabetics have a history of previous malignancy, though this may be due to negative selection, i.e. lower rates of referral or acceptance of patients for dialysis with a history of both diabetes and malignancy.
- **Timing of referral to a nephrologist**. Higher prevalence of vascular disease and malignancy in patients referred late (< 3 months) to a nephrologist.
- **Ethnicity**. Distribution of comorbidity varies according to ethnic group.
  - Diabetes is more common amongst each ethnic minority population than in the White population.
  - The ethnic minority population in the UK is younger than the White population.
- Cause of chronic kidney disease:
  - hypertension;
  - SLE;
  - immunosuppression treatment;
  - previous transplant.

Table 2.1 % new patients with comorbidity starting RRT 1999–2004[1]

	Percentage of patients	
Comorbidity	Age < 65y	Age ≥ 65y
Cardiovascular disease	14.8	32.6
Angina	11.0	24.9
MI in past 3 months	1.8	3.1
MI > 3 months	5.8v	15.5
CABG/angioplasty	4.3	6.6
Cerebrovascular disease	6.4	14.7
Diabetes (not cause of ESRD)	4.9	9.4
Diabetes as primary disease	22.8	16.2
COPD	4.3	10.1
Liver disease	2.5	1.7
Malignancy	6.2	15.5
Peripheral vascular disease	9.4	17.0
Claudication	6.1	13.9
Ischaemic neuropathic ulcers	3.6	3.1
Angioplasty/vascular graft	2.1	4.7
Amputation	2.3	1.7
Smoking	20.8	14.3
No comorbidity present	54.9	35.0

Table 2.2 Percentage of patients with comorbidities amongst South Asian, Afro-Caribbean, and White patients starting RRT 1999–2004[1]

	Percentage of patients of ethnicity		
Comorbidity	South Asian	Black	White
Smoking	7.8	8.4	19.5
CVA	7.3	10.4	11.2
PVD	10.1	4.7	14.3
Cardiovascular disease	24.2	17.5	24.7
Liver disease	4.0	1.4	2.2
COPD	4.3	4.3	8.2
Malignancy	3.2	5.2	12.2

Reference
UK Renal Registry Report 2005.

Diabetes

Diabetes (mainly type 2) is an increasingly common cause of ESRD in all countries, accounting for almost 50% of dialysis patients in some parts of the US, and 20% in Europe. In the UK, percentage of ESRD with diabetes depends on numbers of ethnic minorities, particularly South Asians, living in the catchment area. Patient morbidity and mortality are much worse than for non-diabetic patients as many of the non-renal complications of diabetes will continue to progress after initiation of dialysis.

Macrovascular complications

- **Coronary artery disease**. Present in around a third of diabetic patients starting on dialysis.
  - Presents as angina, acute coronary syndromes, arrhythmias, or sudden death.
  - Complicates haemodialysis because of chest pain, hypotension, and/or arrhythmias during dialysis sessions.
  - Commonly silent; diabetic patients at particular risk of major coronary artery disease with no symptoms of chest pain until a major coronary syndrome or sudden death occurs.
  - Prevents or delays transplantation; coronary investigations essential before transplantation followed by appropriate interventions.
  - Often not amenable to endovascular or surgical treatment.
- **Cerebrovascular disease**. Present in approximately 15% of diabetic patients starting on dialysis.
  - Clinical presentations include transient ischaemic attacks, stroke, vascular dementia.
  - Can be related to carotid artery disease.
  - Potentially a major cause of morbidity.
- **Peripheral vascular disease**. About a quarter of diabetic patients starting on dialysis have PVD.
  - PVD is a major independent predictor of poor outcome on dialysis.
  - Often silent until critical limb ischaemia develops.
  - Often complicated by neuropathy and infection—'the diabetic foot', a major cause of morbidity resulting in:
    — lower limb amputation, often bilateral;
    — upper limb ischaemia, particularly of fingers;
    — severe pain;
    — prolonged hospitalization;
    — difficulty in creating fistulas for vascular access;
    — poor nutrition.

Other complications

- **Retinopathy**. Over 90% patients with type I diabetes and around 80% patients with type II diabetes will have diabetic retinopathy.
  - Patients must continue attending diabetic eye clinics regularly even after starting dialysis.
  - Often patients develop ESRD as a result of poor follow-up and/or management of their diabetes; they are therefore at greatly increased risk of poorly managed diabetic eye disease.

Table 2.3 Percentage of patients with or without diabetes who have comorbid conditions other than diabetes[1]

Comorbidity	Non-diabetics	Diabetics
Coronary artery disease	22.0	30.8
Cerebrovascular disease	9.9	14.8
Peripheral vascular disease	10.4	25.7
Smoking	17.3	18.1
COPD	7.7	5.9
Malignancy	13.2	4.7
Liver disease	2.3	2.0

- Poor vision will have major impact on quality of life.
- Increases chance of being on hospital rather than home dialysis therapy.
- Risk of retinal haemorrhage exacerbated by anticoagulation on HD.
- **Other eye complications**:
  - cataracts;
  - glaucoma: can be extremely painful and may require enucleation of the eye;
  - macular degeneration.
- **Peripheral neuropathy**. This is a major debilitating complication and occurs in the majority of diabetic patients with ESRD:
  - burning pain in the feet that can be very severe;
  - neuropathic ulcers on feet that can become infected: 'diabetic foot';
  - Charcot joints—particularly at ankles;
  - mononeuritis multiplex, i.e. isolated peripheral nerve lesions.
- **Autonomic neuropathy**. Less common than peripheral neuropathy, but occurs more commonly in type 1 diabetics. Causes:
  - postural hypotension; this can be so severe that patients cannot walk without fear of collapsing;
  - impaired bladder functioning with urinary retention;
  - diarrhoea.
- **Gastroparesis**: usually occurs in patients with significant autonomic neuropathy.
  - Can cause severe vomiting.
  - Contributes to poor nutrition.
  - Difficult to treat (see Chapter 7).
- **Infection**. All types more common in diabetic patients. In particular:
  - vascular access infection, particularly of central lines or graft;
  - infection of vascular grafts used for management of PVD;
  - development of osteomyelitis complicates 'diabetic feet'.
- **Sexual dysfunction**. Impotence in men particularly common.

Reference

UK Renal Registry Report 2005.

Cardiovascular disease

Cardiovascular comorbidity is the most common comorbidity in patients with ESRD and is responsible for approximately half of all deaths on dialysis regardless of age, gender, ethnicity, nationality, or primary renal disease. The risk of dying from a myocardial infarct in a 40-year-old man on dialysis is approximately 100-fold greater than the risk for a man of the same age and with normal renal function.

Chronic kidney disease (CKD) and cardiovascular disease (CVD) share many of the same risk factors. It is therefore not surprising that patients with CKD have a greatly increased risk of having CVD and that patients with CVD have a greatly increased risk of having CKD.

Clinically, cardiovascular disease presents as:
- ischaemic heart disease;
- peripheral vascular disease;
- cerebrovascular disease.

Individual patients with any one of these are at greatly increased risk of developing one or both of the others.

Table 2.4 Cardiovascular risk factors in ESRD

General risk factors	Risk factors with increased prevalence in renal failure	Risk factors unique to renal failure
• Age	• Hypertension	• Anaemia
• Male sex	• Diabetes	• Hyperparathyroidism
• Smoking	• Physical inactivity	• Uraemia
• Family history	• Left ventricular hypertrophy	• Hyperphosphataemia
• Thrombogenic factors	• Cholesterol	• Malnutrition
• Obesity	• Lipoproteins(a)	• AV fistulas
	• Homocysteine	• Volume overload
	• Inflammation	• Renal impairment

Ischaemic heart disease

The natural history of ischaemic heart disease in patients with ESRD tends to be more progressive than in the general population. Patients with CKD have an increased mortality after an acute coronary syndrome. Intervention—both coronary angioplasty and coronary artery bypass grafting—also carries a higher mortality risk. Patients with CKD, particularly stages 4 and 5, are much more likely to die, predominantly from ischaemic heart disease, than to eventually require RRT.

Clinical manifestations
- **Exercise-related angina**: similar to patients with normal renal function.
  - Some patients, because of other comorbidities, e.g. PVD, stroke, etc., may not exercise sufficiently to develop chest pain.
  - Exertional dyspnoea and/or arrhythmias may also occur.
- **Angina and/or arrhythmias during dialysis**; commonly associated with episodes of dialysis-related hypotension.
  - Hypotension is more common in patients near their dry weight or in patients with large weight gains between dialyses (so need more fluid removal during dialysis).
  - Development of chest pain on dialysis therefore minimizes fluid removal during dialysis.
  - Patients at risk, therefore, of developing chronic fluid overload resulting in left ventricular dilatation and impaired LV function.
  - Chronic hypotension on and off dialysis develops as a result of impaired LV function. This makes fluid removal on HD even more difficult.
- **Silent myocardial ischaemia** is common in dialysis patients.
  - Patients present with myocardial infarction, serious arrhythmia, or sudden death.
- **Acute myocardial infarction**.
  - Often presents atypically with just shortness of breath or arrhythmias.
  - ECG changes may be difficult to interpret because of pre-existing LVH.
  - Serological diagnosis also more difficult because creatine kinase and troponin T often mildly elevated in patients with ESRD.

Cardiac interventions
Coronary angioplasty + stenting
- Increased risk of complications compared to patients with normal renal function.
- Can achieve better survival than standard medical therapy in selected patients as in general population.
- Can be technically difficult because of calcification of coronary vessels.

Coronary artery bypass grafting
- Typically three or four vessels require grafting.
- Increased postoperative mortality compared to patients without renal disease.

- Increased perioperative morbidity due to wound infection (sternum and vein graft sites), fluid and electrolyte balance related problems, pain control, etc.
- Pre-existing left ventricular dysfunction related to chronic fluid overload increases risk.
- Cardiopulmonary bypass is a major haemodynamic insult that commonly precipitates ESRD in patients with lesser degrees of renal impairment.

Peripheral vascular disease

PVD as a predictor of survival

Analysis of factors affecting survival on dialysis shows that PVD is the worst predictor of outcome

- Most patients with PVD also have other vascular disease, so are at high risk of IHD or cerebrovascular disease.
- More difficult to achieve vascular access for HD.
- Limits chances of successful transplantation as anastamosis on to the iliac artery may be technically difficult or may cause critical limb ischaemia.
- Diagnosis is often made late when critical limb ischaemia has already occurred.
  - Patients may not exercise sufficiently to get claudication, so no warning features.
  - Arteries are often heavily calcified making non-invasive investigations, such as Doppler studies and ankle–brachial pressure ratio, inaccurate as the arteries cannot be compressed.
- Arterial disease is predominantly distal making bypass surgery technically difficult.
- Often associated with poor nutrition.

Clinical features

- Dialysis patients (diabetics and non-diabetics) may present with more diffuse and distal disease compared to those with normal renal function.
- Pre-existing lower limb ischaemia may worsen after creation of permanent HD access in that limb, or after transplantation.
- **Perception of claudication** can vary from severe debilitating discomfort at rest to minor pain of little consequence.
  - Severity of symptoms depends upon amount of stenosis, collateral circulation, and amount of exercise.
  - Location of pain depends upon location of vascular disease. Patients can present with buttock, thigh, calf, or foot claudication.
- **Ischaemic rest pain** typically occurs at night and involves the forefoot and toes. Pain may be more localized in patients who develop an ischaemic ulcer or gangrenous toe.
  - Precipitating factors include trauma superimposed on an area of borderline perfusion.
  - Pain may be relieved by hanging feet over the edge of the bed or walking round the room.
- **Ischaemic neuropathic pain** is related to chronic tissue ischaemia and is described as throbbing or burning often with superimposed severe shooting pains up the limb.
  - Associated with ulcers on lower limb or diabetic foot.

Limb-threatening ischaemia

Limb-threatening ischaemia presents with rest pain, ischaemic ulcers, or gangrene. It usually inexorably progresses to amputation unless arterial perfusion can be improved, e.g. by angioplasty or arterial reconstruction.

- **Rest pain** is brought on or made worse by elevation of the leg and made better by lowering the leg. It is therefore often experienced only at night or when sitting with the legs up.
- **Ischaemic ulcers** are usually dry and are found most commonly at the lateral malleolus, tips of toes, metatarsal heads, and the bunion area.
  - Ischaemic ulcers involving the foot can become infected and lead to osteomyelitis.
- **Gangrene** is characterized by cyanotic, anaesthetic tissue associated with or progressing to necrosis. It can be described as dry or wet.
  - Dry gangrene has a hard and dry texture and commonly occurs at the distal ends of toes and fingers; there is a clear demarcation between viable and necrotic tissue. The involved digit is often allowed to auto-amputate, though this can take a long time.
  - Wet gangrene is an emergency and will often result in amputation.
- **Acute ischaemia** is caused by distal embolization from a proximal atheromatous plaque to digital vessels or occlusion of larger arteries by embolic or thrombotic events. Presentation includes:
  - blue toe syndrome: sudden appearance of cool, painful, cyanotic toe or forefoot often in presence of foot pulses;
  - sudden onset of pain in a limb accompanied by pallor, coolness, and absence of palpable pulses.

Management

- Angioplasty is often not indicated or is not successful as the arterial disease is predominantly distal.
- Management of limb-threatening ischaemia in ESRD patients can be difficult for various reasons:
  - poor wound healing;
  - high rate of infection;
  - poor nutritional state;
  - high operative risk;
  - vascular calcification can make arterial surgery technically difficult.
- Studies show that, after surgical revascularization, patients with ESRD have shorter survival, less subjective improvement, lower limb salvage rates, and lower graft patency compared to non-ESRD patients.
- If revascularization fails or is not technically feasible, amputation of digit, forefoot, or limb is required.

Amputation

Dialysis patients have a very high rate of lower limb amputation compared to the general population.

- Predicted survival is very poor after amputation; reports have been as low as 30% for 2-year survival among Medicare ESRD patients undergoing amputation.
- Prolonged hospitalization often needed after amputation:
  - poor wound healing;
  - difficult pain control;
  - poor nutrition;
  - increased infection risk;
  - slow rehabilitation in patients who frequently have a long history of physical inactivity.
- High risk of developing critical ischaemia in other limb resulting in bilateral amputation.
- Major social aspects and effects on quality of life, particularly after bilateral amputation.
  - If on peritoneal dialysis, may have to transfer to haemodialysis as no longer able to cope with a self-care dialysis modality.
  - Will need assistance with transport to haemodialysis facility.
  - May need rehousing or major changes to accommodation.
  - May no longer be able to live independently and therefore have to transfer to a nursing-home.
  - Prolonged hospitalization with high risk of depression, poor nutrition, social isolation, etc.

Cerebrovascular disease

Stroke is more common in patients with ESRD as hypertension is the major risk factor for cerebrovascular disease.

- Hypotensive episodes on HD can also precipitate cerebrovascular events.
- Patients at most risk are those with poorly controlled hypertension, diabetes, the elderly, smokers, and those with other vascular disease.

Presentation and management
- Presentation is the same as in the general population and includes:
  - transient ischaemic attacks;
  - stroke;
  - multi-infarct dementia.
- Increased risk of haemorrhage into area of cerebral infarction in HD patients using anticoagulation.
- Management of HD can be difficult after a cerebral haemorrhage because of the risk of anticoagulation.
- Transferring a patient to PD (if possible) may avoid further events related to hypotension on dialysis.
- No decision on the long-term outcome should be made immediately, as the prognosis is very variable, as in the general population.
- Important long-term sequelae of stroke in a patient on dialysis include:
  - loss of social independence;
  - difficulty in continuing to perform PD unless there is support from a carer;
  - poor nutrition;
  - depression.

Malignancy

UK Renal Registry data suggest that around 6% patients <65 years old and 15% >65 years old will have a history of malignancy when starting on dialysis. Patients can also develop a new malignancy during their time on RRT. This will obviously have a major impact on individual patients.

> Malignancy is a poor predictor of survival

- Pain control is more complicated in patients with renal disease (see Chapter 6).
- Patients with active malignancy cannot have a renal transplant.
- Management is often more complex than in the general population.
    - Patients with ESRD have a high surgical risk.
    - Many cytotoxic drugs are excreted by the kidneys so their dose has to be altered.
    - Timing of cytotoxic therapy around haemodialysis sessions is often complex.
    - Immunosuppression may have to be reduced in transplant recipients, thereby increasing the risk of rejecting the kidney.
- Patients can become severely malnourished.

Malignancy as cause of renal failure

Several types of malignancy can cause renal failure.

Obstruction to urinary tract
- Bladder outflow obstruction, e.g. Ca prostate, Ca bladder.
- Ureteric obstruction by pelvic tumours, e.g. Ca cervix, Ca rectum.
- Obstruction of ureter of single kidney by transitional cell carcinoma.

Renal tumours requiring bilateral nephrectomy or removal of single functioning kidney:
- can occur de novo in native kidneys; renal cell carcinoma in one kidney increases the likelihood of developing one in the other kidney;
- increased risk of renal cell carcinoma in genetic disorders associated with cystic kidneys, e.g. tuberous sclerosis, von Hippel–Lindau syndrome.

Haematological malignancies can cause ESRD because of renal involvement. Prognosis is related to underlying malignancy and is worse than for patients with ESRD alone and for patients with the malignancy but normal renal function. Examples are:
- myeloma;
- primary amyloid.

Complications of malignancy and/or treatment
- Hypercalcaemia.
- Tumour lysis syndrome.
- Tubular toxins in chemotherapy, e.g. platinum.
- Focal glomerulosclerosis and nephritic syndrome induced by pamidronate.

Coincidental tumours

Patients with ESRD can develop any tumour. The risk of malignancy is increased in ESRD, particularly after renal transplantation, because of reduced immunosurveillance as renal failure is associated with a reduced immune response. The natural history of such tumours is the same as in the general population, with the provisos mentioned at the beginning of this section.

Infection

Various types of infection can cause renal disease and patients with renal disease can have a coincidental infection. In both instances, outcome on ESRD will be affected by the natural history of that infection.

Hepatitis B

- Hepatitis B can cause membranous glomerulonephritis, which can lead to ESRD.
- More commonly, patients with renal disease are carriers of hepatitis B. This is particularly common in:
  - intravenous drug abusers;
  - patients from countries with high prevalence of hepatitis B.
- Many patients with chronic hepatitis B are asymptomatic with a very low risk of cirrhosis or hepatocellular carcinoma.
- Risk of liver damage or carcinoma is increased with immunosuppression, e.g. for treatment of underlying renal disease or transplantation.
- Treatment with antiviral drugs, e.g. lamivudine, may be successful enabling patients to be transplanted.
- Patients who are hepatitis B antigen positive need to be isolated while on HD to prevent transmission of infection to other patients.

Hepatitis C

- Can directly cause renal disease, predominantly membranoproliferative glomerulonephritis associated with cryoglobulinaemia.
- As with hepatitis B, more commonly patients with renal disease are carriers of hepatitis C. This is particularly common in:
  - intravenous drug abusers;
  - patients from countries with high prevalence of hepatitis C.
- Disease has long indolent course but leads to cirrhosis and hepatocellular carcinoma.
- Risk of liver damage or carcinoma is increased with immunosuppression, e.g. for treatment of underlying renal disease or transplantation.
- Treatment with antiviral drugs, e.g. interferon and ribavirin, is associated with more side-effects in patients with renal failure, but may be successful enabling patients to be transplanted.

HIV

- Causes both acute and chronic renal disease; several types of histology are found on renal biopsy.
- Patients can also be carriers of HIV infection; this is particularly common in:
  - intravenous drug abusers;
  - patients from countries with high prevalence of HIV infection, e.g. sub-Saharan Africa;
  - patients with high risk sexual behaviour.
- Use of combination antiretroviral treatment has revolutionized outcome to the extent that patients with negligible viral load are now being given renal transplants.

Tuberculosis
- TB is more common in renal failure and in ethnic minorities most of whom also have an increased incidence of TB.
- Increased risk in patients with HIV.
- Extra-pulmonary involvement is common.
- Should always be considered if unexplained fever not responding to conventional antibiotics.
- Diagnosis often only made by using trial of antituberculous drugs.
- Doses of drugs have to be altered in presence of renal failure.

Complications of end-stage renal disease

Introduction

There are many complications of ESRD as shown in Table 3.1. They can be divided into those directly caused by the abnormal metabolic state of renal failure and those related to the treatment modality used. They contribute significantly to the morbidity and mortality associated with renal disease.

Table 3.1 Complications of renal failure

Metabolic complications	Complications related to RRT
• Uraemia	*Haemodialysis*
• Electrolyte disorders	• Vascular access failure
• Anaemia	• Central venous occlusion
• Fluid overload	• Line infection
• Hypertension	• Dialysis amyloid arthropathy
• Cardiac disease	• Renal cysts & tumours
• Calcium/phosphate regulation	
• Renal bone disease	*Peritoneal dialysis*
• Vascular calcification	• Ultrafiltration failure
• Calciphylaxis	• Peritonitis
• Poor nutrition	• Sclerosing peritonitis
• Neuropathy	
• Vascular disease	*Transplantation*
	• Rejection
	• Infection
	• Malignancy
	• Drug side-effects
	• Cardiovascular disease
	• Osteoporosis
	• Sensitization

Uraemia

Uraemia is the complex of symptoms that develop with severe renal failure; they are summarized in Table 3.2. For patients followed in a renal clinic, RRT (dialysis or pre-emptive transplantation) is commenced before severe uraemic symptoms develop. The level of renal function at which uraemic symptoms appear varies from individual to individual with some complaining of tiredness with GFRs as high as 30mL/min and others denying any symptoms with a GFR as low as 5mL/min. Patients on dialysis often continue to have some uraemic symptoms of varying severity.

More severe uraemic symptoms develop in the following situations.
- When GFR approaches 5mL/min.
- At end of life:
  - patients who opt for conservative care and do not dialyse;
  - patients who discontinue dialysis.
- Underdialysis.

Table 3.2 Uraemic symptoms

Early symptoms start when GFR < 20–30mL/min; become more severe as GFR declines

- Fatigue
- Anorexia
- Pruritis
- Sleep disturbance
- Muscle cramps
- Feeling cold

Late symptoms start when GFR < 10mL/min

- Nausea and vomiting
- Lethargy, apathy
- Weight loss
- Peripheral oedema & dyspnoea
- Pulmonary oedema
- Nocturia & polyuria
- Bleeding tendency
- Metabolic flap
- Myoclonic jerks
- Restless legs

Symptoms towards end of life start when GFR ~5mL/min

- Neuropathy
- Proximal myopathy
- Severe pruritis (sometimes with skin excoriation)
- Pericarditis
- Fits
- Cognitive impairment
- Confusion
- Coma

Electrolyte disorders

The most common electrolyte disorders found in patients with ESRD are:
- hyperkalaemia;
- hypokalaemia;
- hyponatraemia.

Hyperkalaemia

The causes of high plasma potassium in patients with ESRD include the following.
- Dietary intake from, e.g. fruit, vegetables, chocolate.
- Underdialysis.
- Drugs:
  - ACE inhibitors or A2 receptor blockers;
  - spironolactone;
  - potassium supplements.
- Breakdown of blood products releasing potassium from red cells:
  - blood transfusion;
  - gastrointestinal bleeding;
  - absorption of blood from a haematoma.
- Metabolic acidosis (see below).

Symptoms
- Often none.
- Cardiac arrhythmia—ventricular or atrial.
- Cardiac arrest.
- GI symptoms—abdominal pain, diarrhoea.

Hypokalaemia

Low plasma potassium is less common.
- Usually associated with poor nutrition, and therefore low potassium intake.
- Can occur in patients on high doses of loop diuretics, e.g. furosemide, bumetanide for fluid control:
  - predialysis or conservative care patients;
  - peritoneal dialysis;
  - transplant with poor function.
- Increased risk of cardiac arrhythmias particularly in patients on HD.
- Can exacerbate symptoms of fatigue and lethargy.

Hyponatraemia

Low plasma sodium is not uncommon in patients on dialysis or with ESRD.
- Usually associated with fluid overload with proportionally more water than sodium in extracellular fluid.
- Occurs in patients with high water intake and poor oral intake of sodium.
- Increases symptoms of fatigue, lethargy, nausea, confusion.

Anaemia

Anaemia

Anaemia is universal in ESRD primarily due to a relative lack of erythropoietin (EPO). There is a strong association between Hb and risk of death in ESRD. Increasing Hb causes major improvements in many uraemic symptoms including exercise capacity, cognitive function, nutrition, sleep patterns. Around 80–90% patients on dialysis will require EPO and iron therapy to maintain their Hb in the range of 11–12g/dL.

Erythropoietin resistance

This is common at end of life and is related to many of the problems common at this time.
- Concurrent infection/inflammation.
- Hyperparathyroidism.
- Malignancy.
- Malnutrition.
- Inadequate dialysis.
- Bone marrow disorders, e.g. myelodysplasia.
- Blood loss.

Difficulty in treating anaemia and therefore failure to achieve Hb targets will result in:
- increased fatigue;
- anorexia;
- worsening of heart failure;
- increased ischaemic symptoms, e.g. angina, claudication;
- increased dependence on blood transfusions.
  - Red cell antibodies are reasonably common in these patients increasing the difficulty in obtaining blood.

Fluid overload

Fluid overload is, not surprisingly, a common problem in ESRD patients and can cause significant distress with shortness of breath at the end of life. Various factors contribute to its development.

- Difficulty in restricting fluid intake.
- Inadequate fluid removal on dialysis:
  - poor ultrafiltration and loss of residual renal function on peritoneal dialysis;
  - difficulty with vascular access for haemodialysis;
  - hypotensive episodes on HD requiring infusion of saline thereby making fluid removal difficult.

Oedema associated with fluid overload also causes problems:
- impaired healing of ischaemic or venous ulcers;
- increased risk of cellulitis.

Vicious circle of heart failure and fluid overload

Chronic fluid overload results in left ventricular dilatation with resulting poor cardiac function and hypotension, which then increases the difficulty of removing fluid on dialysis.

Calcium/phosphate disorders

Hyperparathyroidism

- Hyperparathyroidism is the key to calcium and phosphate disorders in renal disease.
- Primary cause is failure of the kidney to synthesize 1,25 dihydroxy vitamin D_3 (calcitriol), which is the active metabolite of vitamin D.
- As a result, intestinal calcium absorption is reduced leading to hypocalcaemia which stimulates parathyroid hormone secretion.
- The raised PTH acts on the bones releasing calcium and phosphate and thereby restoring plasma calcium levels towards normal but at the expense of hyperphosphataemia.

Hyperphosphataemia

Phosphate levels are an independent predictor of survival on dialysis and start rising when GFR falls below 30mL/min/1.73m^2. Factors determining phosphate levels include:
- level of residual renal function;
- dietary intake of phosphate;
- degree of secondary hyperparathyroidism;
- use of vitamin D metabolites, e.g. calcitriol, alfacalcidol;
- dialysis adequacy;
- dose of phosphate binders (and compliance with their use).

Renal bone disease

All patients with ESRD have renal bone disease by the time they require dialysis, though of varying severity. Dialysis is not a cure but merely a prolongation of the state of renal failure. Renal bone disease therefore progresses and is not cured when patients are on dialysis.

Clinical features

Symptoms do not develop until an advanced stage of renal bone disease, and often patients do not complain of bone pains unless specifically asked, or after suppression of raised PTH by parathyroidectomy or treatment with cinacalcet (a calcimimetic). Symptoms can be divided into different groups.
- Related to calcium phosphate metabolism:
  - pruritis (calcium phosphate deposition under the skin);
  - soft tissue calcification leading to tender lumps under the skin;
  - calcification of tendons leading to acute joint problems;
  - symptoms of hypercalcaemia if present (i.e. nausea, vomiting, constipation, confusion).
- Related to bone pathology:
  - joint pains—often widespread and only commented on by patients when hyperparathyroidism treated;
  - bone pains;
  - fractures—particularly of pelvis with vitamin D deficiency (osteomalacia).
- Related to raised PTH level:
  - mild depression.

Contributing factors to renal bone disease

- Hyperparathyroidism
- Acidosis
- Low vitamin D levels (in certain groups of patients)
- Suppressed parathyroid activity (after treatment)
- Aluminium accumulation (now rare)
- Osteoporosis in elderly patients
- Osteopenia caused by steroids used to treat initial disease or for transplantation

Vascular calcification

- Common in ESRD.
- Can be very obvious on plain X-rays, which may look like an arteriogram.
- Important underlying factor causing cardiovascular disease in patients with ESRD.
- Includes heart valves.
- Multiple predisposing factors:
  - hyperparathyroidism;
  - hyperphosphataemia;
  - inflammation;
  - calcium loading from calcium-containing phosphate binders (calcium carbonate, calcium lactate), particularly in the presence of oversuppressed parathyroid glands (low turnover bone disease).

Calciphylaxis

- A syndrome of vascular calcification and skin necrosis occurring rarely in patients with ESRD.
- Associated with hypercalcaemia, hyperphosphataemia, hyperparathyroidism, vitamin D treatment, and IV iron, but precise cause unknown.
- High mortality (60–80%); mostly from sepsis from infected necrotic skin.
- Lesions are very painful, occur usually on legs, develop suddenly, and progress rapidly.
  - Start as erythematous papules; then become necrotic or even bullous.
- Commoner proximally on thighs, buttocks, and lower abdomen, but can occur distally.
- Vascular calcification is a constant feature, but distal pulses are usually present.

Poor nutrition

Over a third of patients with ESRD are malnourished. This is associated with increased infection, poor wound healing, muscle wasting, and increased mortality. Poor nutritional status prior to initiation of dialysis is also associated with poorer outcomes on dialysis and increased mortality. Malnutrition is caused by inadequate dietary intake or unmet increased nutritional requirements.

Diagnosing malnutrition

- Clinical features:
  - weight loss;
  - muscle wasting;
  - anorexia;
  - fatigue on exercise.
- Biochemical features:
  - reduction in plasma creatinine over time indicating reduction in muscle mass;
  - low plasma urea (< 15mmol/L) indicating inadequate protein intake;
  - hypokalaemia suggesting poor nutritional intake as potassium is found in wide range of foods;
  - hypophosphataemia also indicates overall poor food intake;
  - low plasma cholesterol.

Consequences of poor nutrition

- Increased risk of infection.
- Anorexia, nausea.
- Low plasma albumin.
- Oedema associated with hypoalbuminaemia.
- Muscle fatigue—reduced exercise tolerance.
- Depression.
- Feeling cold.
- Increased mortality.

Factors causing malnutrition in ESRD

Factors increasing nutrient requirements
- Metabolic abnormalities
  - Metabolic acidosis
  - Inflammation—increased cytokine activity
  - Leptin activity
- Concomitant disease
  - Cardiovascular disease
  - Sepsis
  - MIA syndrome: malnutrition, inflammation, atherosclerosis

Factors decreasing food intake
- Anorexia
  - Nausea, fatigue, taste changes, anaemia
- GI disturbances
  - Phosphate binders, antibiotics, uraemic & diabetic gastroparesis
- Psychosocial & socioeconomic
  - Depression, anxiety, ignorance, loneliness, alcohol or drug abuse, poverty

Neuropathy

A peripheral polyneuropathy develops in advanced renal failure or in patients who are underdialysed. It is more common in men and affects mostly the lower limbs.

Clinical manifestations

- Sensory symptoms (paraesthesiae, burning sensations, pain) occur before motor symptoms.
- Sensory symptoms improve rapidly on starting or increasing dialysis.
- Motor involvement resulting in muscle atrophy, myoclonus, and eventual paralysis is not reversible.

Sensory syndromes

- Restless leg syndrome—a persistent and uncomfortable sensation in lower extremities that can only be relieved by movement of the legs.
  - More prominent at night and may interfere with sleep.
- Burning foot syndrome—severe pain and burning sensation in distal lower extremities.
  - Can be due to thiamine deficiency as this vitamin is water soluble and well dialysed.
- Paradoxical heat sensation—application of low temperature stimuli evokes sensation of high temperature.

Complications of haemodialysis

Vascular access failure

Vascular access is the Achilles heel of haemodialysis; without it patients cannot be put on HD. The various types of access used include the following.

- Native arteriovenous fistulas. Choices of location (in order of preference) are:
  - radiocephalic (wrist);
  - radiobasilic (wrist);
  - brachiocephalic (elbow);
  - brachiobasilic transposition (involves freeing and transposition of basilica vein);
  - thigh.
- Prosthetic grafts, usually using Goretex:
  - upper arm;
  - thigh.
- Tunnelled central venous catheters:
  - jugular vein;
  - subclavian vein.

The complications of all types of access are predominantly thrombosis and infection. These occur less frequently with native AV fistulas, but these fistulas are less likely to be successful in patients with vascular disease. After the standard sites have been used or if they are not feasible, various other access sites can be used:

- grafts connecting distant arteries and veins, e.g. across the chest from axillary artery to vein, or from axillary artery to femoral vein;
- central venous catheters placed into femoral or lumbar veins.

These various access procedures have much higher failure rates, are more likely to thrombose, and are therefore unlikely to last longer than a few months.

Central venous occlusion

Catheterization of any central vein can result in occlusion of that vein when the catheter is removed, even in the absence of infection or catheter thrombosis. The clinical consequences of this include:

- loss of that vein for future access;
- loss of ipsilateral arm for future AV fistula formation (particularly with subclavian vein thrombosis) because of reduced venous return;
- swollen arm if central venous occlusion occurs with functioning AV fistula because of high venous pressure;
- swollen face and neck if bilateral central venous occlusion;
- dilated veins across anterior chest wall;
- swollen leg from femoral vein thrombosis with risk of pulmonary embolus.

Line infection Bacteraemia is a major complication of the use of central venous catheters for HD. It is more common with temporary catheters but not insignificant when using tunnelled lines. Complications include:

- need to remove catheter (and therefore loss of vascular access) if temperature does not settle within 2–3 days of starting antibiotics, or if recurrent infection;
- endocarditis, particularly in patients with pre-existing valvular disease;
- discitis with epidural abscess and resulting paraplegia (fortunately rare);
- embolic abscess formation at other sites, e.g. joints.

Dialysis amyloid arthropathy

This is a complication of long-term dialysis and becomes increasingly more common after 10 years; it is due to β2-microglobulin amyloidosis. The incidence of this complication has reduced with improvement in biocompatibility of dialysis membranes.

Clinical features

- Carpal tunnel occurs first. Most patients who been on dialysis more than 20 years are affected and will have needed surgery; usually affects both hands.
- Joint pains and stiffness, usually bilateral, starting in the shoulders and extending to other joints. Pain is often worse at night and during HD.
- As the disease progresses, joint movements become restricted, particularly the shoulders.
- Chronic tenosynovitis of the finger flexors causes restricted movement, pain, and trigger fingers. Can become incapacitating.
- Very rarely, extra-articular accumulation of amyloid results in lumps, e.g. in the tongue or subcutaneously near joints.
- Destructive spondylarthropathy usually of the cervical spine.
- Rarely, amyloid may be deposited in the epidural space causing spinal cord compression.
- Pathological fractures, particularly of the femoral neck, due to amyloid cysts weakening the bone.

Renal cysts and tumours

- *Renal cysts* are common in patients on dialysis. They are usually asymptomatic. The important associated clinical features are:
  - haemorrhage into the retroperitoneal space—this can be life-threatening and can cause significant hyperkalaemia;
  - erythropoietin production; patients may no longer need exogenous erythropoietin administration and can become polycythaemic;
  - risk of malignancy (see below).
- *Renal tumours* (predominantly renal carcinomas) are more common in patients with ESRD, particularly those on dialysis.
- Predominantly a complication of long-term dialysis with increasing frequency after 10 years.
- Mostly associated with cystic kidneys and can present with retroperitoneal haemorrhage.
- Often no symptoms until presenting with metastases.

Complications of peritoneal dialysis

Ultrafiltration failure

Ultrafiltration is key to the success of PD, particularly once patients have become anuric. The methods used to increase ultrafiltration include the use of hypertonic dextrose dialysate, use of icodextrin (a glucose polymer), and use of APD in patients who have rapid transport membrane characteristics. As the peritoneal membrane transport tends to become more rapid with time on PD, some long-term PD patients develop ultrafiltration failure. They are then at risk of developing fluid overload and ideally should discontinue PD and transfer to HD.

Peritonitis

Peritonitis is a major cause of morbidity in patients on PD. The overall peritonitis rate in most units is 1 in 20–30 patient months. Some patients seem never to get peritonitis, while others have recurrent episodes. This can be due to patient technique, particularly with Gram-positive infections (*Staphylococcus epidermidis* and *Staphylococcus aureus*). Gram-negative infections are often associated with underlying bowel disease, and are therefore more common in elderly patients because of the presence of diverticular disease.

Clinical features
- Abdominal pain.
- Cloudy fluid.
- Fever in more severe cases.
- 80% cure rate with intraperitoneal antibiotics.

Complications
- Failure to respond to treatment necessitating catheter removal.
  - More common with Gram-negative infections.
  - Patient then needs urgent transfer to HD with central venous catheter (unless pre-existing fistula).
- *Clostridium difficile* infection as a consequence of using broad-spectrum antibiotics for treatment of peritonitis.
- Worsening nutrition because of increased peritoneal protein losses.

Predictors of peritonitis
- Poor patient technique:
  - social issues, e.g. housing;
  - cognitive problems;
  - depression.
- Exit site and tunnel infection.
- Active bowel disease, e.g. diverticulitis.
- PD being done in hospital:
  - patient unwell so not so careful with technique;
  - nurses often inexperienced at PD particularly if high turnover and not receiving regular education about technique.

Encapsulating peritoneal sclerosis

This is also known as sclerosing peritonitis. Encapsulating peritoneal sclerosis (EPS) is a devastating complication of long-term PD. Prevalence is ~2% in patients on PD for 3–5 years and 20% in patients on PD for more than 8 years. The condition consists of a thick-walled membranous cocoon that wraps itself round loops of bowel causing intestinal obstruction and subsequent malnutrition.

Clinical course

- Symptoms of full-blown EPS are:
  - vomiting;
  - abdominal pain;
  - intermittent small bowel obstruction;
  - ascites—often massive; can be haemorrhagic.
- Clinical symptoms of bowel obstruction more commonly occur when patients stop doing PD. Thus patients can appear well on PD but develop the syndrome within a short time (sometimes only weeks) of transplantation or transferring to HD.
- Course can be more insidious with symptoms developing after several months or even year or two after transferring to HD.
- Can be precipitated by episode of peritonitis even early in the time span of PD.
- There is no proven treatment, though steroids, immunosuppressive drugs, and surgery are all occasionally used. Some patients appear to respond to tamoxifen, which has anti-fibrotic actions, but there is no randomized trial to support this observation. At least, tamoxifen has no major side-effects.
- Mortality is high with 50% of patients with EPS dying within a few months of diagnosis, usually from malnutrition.

Complications of transplantation

1-year graft survival rates of 90–95% are now readily achievable for first grafts with the use of current immunosuppression regimes. Transplantation is therefore being offered to more 'marginal' candidates, i.e. older individuals, diabetics, and patients with ischaemic heart disease once it has been treated with angioplasty or surgery. Although the number of cadaveric organs is not rising, a dramatic increase in transplantation rates is being achieved by encouragement of living donor transplantation, often from unrelated donors, particularly spouses. In many UK units, over 50% of new transplants are from living donors. It is not surprising that, with an older recipient population, there is a higher rate of complications.

Rejection

Acute rejection is now relatively rare. Most transplants are lost during the first year because of surgical complications. Chronic rejection is the most common cause of graft failures after the first year. This is an incompletely understood process, which is also known by various other names such as transplant glomerulopathy or chronic renal allograft nephropathy.

- Clinical diagnosis is suggested by slowly rising plasma creatinine, increasing proteinuria, and worsening hypertension.
- Important to rule out transplant artery stenosis causing deterioration in renal function.
- Changing immunosuppression may have some effect on slowing down rate of progression.
- Important to control BP and cholesterol as some of damage is due to progressive glomerulosclerosis.
- At risk of developing other complications of ESRD, e.g. anaemia, hyperparathyroidism, as renal function deteriorates.
- Over 25–30% people on waiting lists for a renal transplant have had one or more previous transplants.

Infection

Infection is a problem at all time points after transplantation.

- There is an increased risk of all types of infection, including:
  - common, community-acquired bacteria and viruses;
  - TB particularly in those from at risk ethnic groups, e.g. South Asian;
  - uncommon opportunistic infections that occur only in immunocompromised individuals, e.g. pneumocystis, nocardia, aspergillus, CMV, etc.
- Urinary tract infection. Major risk factors are:
  - indwelling bladder catheters;
  - handling and trauma to kidney and ureter during surgery;
  - anatomic abnormalities of native or transplanted kidneys (e.g. reflux, stones, or stents);
  - neurogenic bladder.
- Chronic viral infections. These can have either caused the kidney disease, or patient may be a carrier.
  - Hepatitis B.
  - Hepatitis C.
  - HIV.

Malignancy

Post-transplant lymphoproliferative disorders (PTLD) are the most common malignancy complicating the chronic immunosuppression used for transplantation.

- More than 50% patients with PTLD present with extranodal masses, e.g. in stomach, lungs, skin, liver, CNS, and allograft itself.
- Around 25% will have CNS disease.
- Involvement of transplanted kidney can result in renal failure.
- Principal risk factors are degree of overall immunosuppression and Epstein–Barr virus status of the recipient.
- Incidence is highest in first year when immunosuppression dosage is at its highest
- Reducing immunosuppression increases risk of rejection but, if done carefully, can result in a high response rate and low rate of rejection.
- Can also be treated with chemotherapy and radiotherapy.
- Mortality can be high with rates up to 80% reported.

Skin cancers post-transplantation Chronic immunosuppression is associated with increased incidence of skin cancers.

- Squamous cell carcinomas occur over a 100 times more commonly in transplant patients, with the highest risk in patients with a history of high sun exposure.
- Incidence of basal cell carcinoma is increased 10-fold.
- Skin cancers are often multiple and more than one type can occur in the same patient.

Skin tumours are more aggressive and are more likely to recur after resection in patients with transplants than in the general population.

Solid tumours particularly squamous cell carcinomas are more common in transplant recipients because of reduced immunosurveillance. Compared with the incidence in the general population, the following tumours particularly are more common in transplant recipients:

- Kaposi's sarcoma;
- non-Hodgkin's lymphoma;
- renal cell cancer;
- vulvovaginal cancer.

Immunosuppression drug side-effects

All immunosuppressive drugs have side-effects other than those related to the immunosuppression itself.

Steroids

- Cushingoid appearance.
- Obesity.
- Diabetes.
- Thin skin with easy bruising.
- Poor wound healing.
- Hypertension.

- Bone disease:
  - osteoporosis;
  - osteopenia;
  - avascular necrosis.
- Gastric erosions.

Cyclosporin

- Diabetes.
- Hypertension.
- Nephrotoxicity.
- Drug interactions due to metabolism by cytochrome P450 enzymes in the liver.
  - Drugs causing raised cyclosporin levels include diltiazem, fluconazole, erythromycin, lansoprazole, cimetidine, allopurinol.
  - Drugs causing decreased cyclosporin levels include rifampicin, phenytoin, orlistat.
- Hirsutism.
- Gingival hyperplasia and gingivitis.
- Tremor.
- Metabolic abnormalities:
  - hyperkalaemia;
  - hyperuricaemia and gout.
- Bone disease—increased bone turnover leading to bone loss.

Tacrolimus

- Not as well studied as cyclosporin, but range of side-effects is very similar.
- Early studies suggested that diabetes is more common than with cyclosporin, but this is probably not so when mycophenylate given as well.

Azathioprine

- Bone marrow suppression.
- Skin malignancies.

Mycophenylate

- Diarrhoea.
- Hypertension.
- Peripheral oedema.
- Insomnia.

Sirolimus

- Bone marrow suppression.
- Raised cholesterol and triglycerides.
- Diarrhoea or constipation.
- Haemolytic uraemic syndrome when used in combination with cyclosporin.
- Interstitial pneumonitis; this is reversible on withdrawing sirolimus.

- Skin problems are common:
  - delayed wound healing;
  - acne;
  - scalp folliculitis;
  - oedema;
  - aphthous ulceration.

Cardiovascular disease

Risk of CVD after renal transplantation is reduced compared to the risk in patients on dialysis. This is only partly due to the fact that patients are screened for CVD and/or appropriately treated (e.g. with stents or surgery) before transplantation. CVD, nevertheless, remains much more common in transplant recipients than in the normal population and is the most common cause of death in transplant recipients.

Factors contributing to CVD in transplant recipients include:
- hypertension;
- diabetes;
- obesity;
- pre-existing CVD;
- length of time on dialysis pre-transplantation;
- deteriorating renal function post-transplantation;
- immunosuppressive drugs—steroids, cyclosporin, tacrolimus (see above);
- physical inactivity.

Bone disease

Osteopenia and bone fractures are common after transplantation.
- Rapid bone loss occurs in first 6 months after transplantation.
- Patients start life with a transplant with hyperparathyroid bone disease or low turnover bone metabolism from overtreated hyperparathyroidism.
- Steroids and cyclosporin/tacrolimus contribute to bone loss (see above).
- Acidosis related to poor renal function and/or use of cyclosporin contributes to altered bone metabolism.

Sensitization

Patients are at risk of developing HLA antibodies after a failed transplant.
- It is important to avoid same HLA antigens in subsequent transplants. This makes matching more difficult and therefore may entail a longer wait for a kidney.
- Patients can become sensitized to a broad range of antigens, particularly if given blood transfusions. This can make it very difficult to find suitable donors.

Causes of death in end-stage renal disease

Mortality

Mortality rates for patients with ESRD are worse than for most cancers with an overall median survival of less than 6 years, though this does vary with age. UK Renal Registry data[1] shows that 5-year survival after starting RRT is:
- > 90% for 18–34 year olds;
- 70% for 45–54 year olds;
- 30% for 65–74 year olds;
- < 20% for > 75 year olds.

These rates are much lower than in the general population. The mortality rate for 45–54 year olds is about 18 times that for people of the same age in the general population. This is also true for the elderly: mortality rate for > 75 year olds is about 4-fold higher.

Predictors of increased mortality risk

Having one or more of the comorbidities or complications mentioned in Chapters 2 and 3 will increase the risk of morbidity and mortality. The list below summarizes some of these. These various factors do, however, interrelate so multivariate analyses in most studies show that the key predictors of poor survival are age, comorbidity, and poor nutrition. Predictors of increased mortality include the following.
- Being on dialysis compared to having a functioning transplant.
- Age.
- Vascular comorbidity.
  - Peripheral vascular disease has been shown to be the most important predictor of poor survival in many studies.
  - Ischaemic heart disease.
  - Cerebrovascular disease.
- Diabetes.
- Poor nutrition.
- Malignancy.
- Low plasma albumin.
- Poor control of calcium and phosphate levels:
  - hyperphosphataemia;
  - hypercalcaemia;
  - raised calcium–phosphate product.
- Impaired cardiac function:
  - left ventricular hypertrophy;
  - left ventricular dilatation;
  - hypotension.
- Anaemia:
  - erythropoietin resistance.
- Infection:
  - chronic viral infections, e.g. hepatitis B, C, HIV;
  - recurrent dialysis-related infections.
- Poor compliance.
- Poor vascular access.

- Lack of predialysis renal care.
  - 30–40% patients are referred less than 1 month before needing to start dialysis—so-called crash landers.
  - Mortality rate for such patients increased by 15–30% in several studies.
  - Detrimental effects of late referral are summarized in the box.

Detrimental effects of late referral

- Lack of interventions that might slow progression of renal failure
- Failure to plan for RRT
- Failure to plan vascular access with consequent increased reliance on central venous catheters and risk of infection
- Failure to provide psychological and social support
- Increased hospitalization rate
- Lower quality of life

Reference
UK Renal Registry Report 2005.

Causes of death

Causes of death are related to pre-existing comorbidity and complications of ESRD.

Cardiac causes

> Cardiac causes account for over 50% of deaths

- Myocardial infarction accounts for less than 10% of these deaths.
- Heart failure with left ventricular dilatation is more common—often related to chronic fluid overload.
- About 60% of cardiac deaths are sudden due to arrhythmias related to electrolyte disorders or impaired cardiac function.

Peripheral vascular disease

- Amputation.
- Sepsis—gangrene, osteomyelitis.
- Often associated with poor nutrition.
- Associated cardiac disease.

Cerebrovascular disease

- Stroke.
- Complications of stroke—poor nutrition, depression.
- Associated cardiac disease.

Infection accounts for around 20% of deaths.
- General infections, e.g. pneumonia.
- Dialysis-related—septicaemia (HD), peritonitis (PD).
- Transplant-related—general + opportunistic infections.

Malignancy
- One-sixth less common than cardiac disease.
- More common in transplant recipients.

Stopping dialysis Usually in association with one or more of the above.

Cardiac arrest

Causes

Sudden death has many causes and cannot be simply ascribed to 'cardiac' causes:

- large electrolyte swings (particularly potassium);
- volume overload;
- arrhythmias;
- aortic dissection;
- intracerebral haemorrhage;
- subdural haematoma;
- cerebrovascular disease;
- infection.

Outcome of cardiac arrest

Commonly occurs on dialysis unit as well as outside the hospital. This raises issues of cardiopulmonary resuscitation (CPR), and 'do not resuscitate' orders, which should be discussed in advance with patients and their families. A number of studies have looked at outcome of cardiac arrest in dialysis patients.

- Outcome worse than in general population: only 8% of resuscitated dialysis patients leave hospital compared to 12% of general population
- In one study, 80% of patients who initially responded to CPR were dead within 4 days
- Patients and families have a much more optimistic attitude towards CPR. Education and advanced planning are therefore important

Stopping dialysis

UK Renal Registry data[1] show that up to 25% of deaths in patients on dialysis is due to withdrawal of treatment, particularly in older patients. In the majority of instances, this decision is made when death is close and inevitable. Less commonly, a patient may decide to stop dialysis because of a gradual decline in their health. Examples of both are given in the box.

Suggestion of dialysis withdrawal is often made by the physician but is also commonly made by the patient or a family member. Frequently the patient may make the request to their dialysis nurse or a nurse on the ward rather than to a doctor directly. Such requests should be followed up with discussions with medical staff, counsellors, social workers, and the family. See Chapters 11 and 12.

Time to death after dialysis withdrawal depends on coexisting illness and residual renal function. Death will usually occur within 2 days in the presence of severe illness. In patients established on HD, time to death after stopping dialysis is a median of 8–9 days in almost all studies. Some can survive longer if there is significant residual renal function. This is more common in patients who have only recently started dialysis.

Withdrawal of dialysis

Patient 1

SS was an 86-year-old man who had been on peritoneal dialysis for 5 years. He originally had coped very well but over the years became more short of breath because of underlying chronic obstructive airways disease. It became increasingly difficult for him and his wife to cope with dialysis at home, and, a year before he died, an attempt was made to change to haemodialysis. He tolerated this very poorly and had a cardiac arrest on the second dialysis. The family therefore decided to continue with peritoneal dialysis at home. One year later he was admitted with a gangrenous leg. He was in severe pain, hypotensive, and confused. After discussions with the medical team, the wife and son felt he would not want to go ahead with an amputation. Dialysis was stopped and he died peacefully 2 days later.

Patient 2

Julia was a 35-year-old woman who had been on peritoneal dialysis for 8 years following haemolytic uraemic syndrome associated with pregnancy. The first 5 years had gone well. Julia had managed to work as a teacher and accompany her husband when he travelled for work to Europe. Having initially been not keen on transplantation, she then accepted a kidney from her husband. Unfortunately, this failed immediately because of renal vein thrombosis. She subsequently continued on peritoneal dialysis but accepted she would have to convert to haemodialysis as she was losing ultrafiltration. However, three attempts at fistula formation failed.

One weekend she was admitted with her first episode of peritonitis. This failed to resolve and the catheter had to be removed. At laparatomy extensive fibrous adhesions were found between the bowel loops and a diagnosis of encapsulating peritoneal sclerosis (EPS) was made. Haemodialysis, however, did not go well; catheters only lasted a few days because of clotting problems. She also had continuous abdominal pain and was going to need parenteral nutrition as she did not tolerate any oral fluids. Although her prognosis was poor, there was a possibility that, with parenteral nutrition and eventual formation of definitive vascular access, she would be able to leave hospital, though after a prolonged admission. After many discussions with the healthcare team, she decided that she would rather discontinue dialysis when her current venous access failed. This happened during the next dialysis. Treatment was then stopped and she was given appropriate pain relief and eventually sedation. She died a week later.

Reference

UK Renal Registry Report 2005.

Conservative care

With increasing awareness of the poor outcome on dialysis for older patients with multiple comorbidities, the option of no dialysis is increasingly becoming a standard component of predialysis education. Around 8% of the predialysis patients in London select conservative management.

Conservative management

It is important that patients continue to be actively managed, even when they decide that dialysis is not for them.

- Survival depends on renal function and comorbidity; median survival once GFR is < 10mL/min is around 8 months.
- Correction of anaemia with erythropoietin improves symptoms and quality of life.
- Correction of hypocalcaemia to prevent fits.
- Use of diuretics to prevent pulmonary oedema.
- Appropriate referral to community services and palliative care.
- Re-offering option of dialysis when patients become more symptomatic.

Causes of death

- Often patients will die from their comorbid diseases, e.g. cardiac or vascular disease, malignancy.
- Death will also occur from uraemia.
  - Increasing drowsiness and confusion.
  - Coma.
  - Arrhythmia related to hyperkalaemia causing sudden death.
  - Pulmonary oedema.

See also Chapter 12.

Conservative care

Patient 1

Mr M was a 78-year-old man who was being followed in the renal clinic with CKD and hypertension. He had never married and lived with his nephew. During an admission with an acute coronary syndrome, he decided he did not want active cardiac treatment or dialysis when needed. At that time his plasma creatinine was 350µmol/L and Hb 8.2g/dL. On discharge, he was started on erythropoietin treatment and his Hb was subsequently maintained around 12g/dL. Over the next 2 years he was reasonably well and lived independently; plasma creatinine continued to rise but slowly and reached 450µmol/L. He continued to state that he did not want dialysis when needed. 2 years after the initial coronary event, he was again admitted with severe chest pain and hypotension. On discussion, he stated that he did not want resuscitation if needed. He died from a cardiac arrest 2 days later.

Patient 2

Mr C was an 85-year-old man who was referred to the renal physicians having had a fit in the urology clinic that he was attending for management of urinary retention. He was a practising Scientologist and had resisted referral to hospital until he went into acute retention. Blood results showed creatinine 834µmol/L; urea 45mmol/L; Ca 1.5mmol/L; phosphate 2.6mmol/L; potassium 5.6mmol/L; Hb 5.2g/dL. Renal ultrasound showed two small kidneys. Discussions were held with him and his wife. Both were adamant that they did not want dialysis. He was started on erythropoietin treatment and given supplies of alfacalcidol and calcium supplements but he did not take them. He continued to have intermittent fits and generally deteriorated. His wife was also elderly and fairly frail and could not nurse him at home. At the end, he was admitted to hospital where he gradually went into coma and died 2 days later.

Health-related quality of life in end-stage renal disease

Introduction

'The quality, not the longevity, of one's life is what is important'

Dr Martin Luther King, Jr

Quality of life has many definitions; it is a concept that relates to an overall sense of an individual's well-being. It includes an individual's satisfaction with their life and relates to their ability to take pleasure in everyday activities. Health-related quality of life (HRQL) extends this definition to include the way a person's health affects their ability to carry out normal social and physical activities.

In the last 15 years there has been an increase in studies that measure the HRQL in ESRD patients using standard measures such as the generic Medical Outcomes Study Short Form-36 (SF-36) or the renal specific Kidney Disease Quality of Life Questionnaire (KDQOL). Most of these studies, such as the study of 18 000 RRT patients in 2000,[1] compare HRQL of patients on different modalities of RRT. There are, however, no randomized controlled trials of different treatment modalities with HRQL measurements. Within these limitations it appears that overall there is similar physical HRQL in both HD and PD patients with a trend towards better mental HRQL in PD patients, though home HD patients reported better HRQL in the UK study. There are no studies that compare quality of life for patients on dialysis with those who choose the conservative pathway where the comparison is between groups with similar comorbidity and performance status, or for those in the months leading up to dialysis compared with when dialysis is established.

HRQL and mortality

Poor HQRL has been shown to be a predictor of poor outcome in both American and European studies. This data is insufficiently robust to form the basis for treatment decisions; however, formal measurement of HRQL taken in conjunction with clinical factors contributes to treatment choices for clinicians and patients.

HRQL and the elderly

Quality of life decisions are particularly important when considering dialysis in the elderly or those of any age with multiple and disabling comorbidity. The HRQL of an elderly UK dialysis group was compared with that of a similar group who did not have renal failure needing dialysis and, although physical HRQL was impaired in the dialysis group in comparison with the control group, there was no difference in mental HRQL component.[2] Measures of quality of life used in such studies give useful in-formation for the population studied, but do not tell us how individual patients cope with their disease.

HRQL and pain and other symptoms

Davison and colleagues have shown that there is a correlation between symptom burden and HRQL as well as a statistically significant difference in quality of life scores between those who have moderate to severe pain compared to those with none or mild pain.[3,4]

References

1 Diaz-Buxo JA, Lowrie EG, Lew NL, et al. (2000). Quality of life evaluation using Short Form 36; comparison in haemodialysis and peritoneal dialysis patients. *Am J Kidney Dis* **35**, 293–300.

2 Lamping DL, Constantinovici N, Roderick P, et al. (2000). Clinical outcomes, quality of life and costs from the North Thames Dialysis Study of elderly people on dialysis: a prospective cohort study. *Lancet* **356**, 1543–50.

3 Davison SN, JJhangri GS, Johnson JA (2006). Longitudinal validation of a modified Edmonton symptom assessment system (ESAS) in haemodialysis patients. *Nephrol Dial Transplant* **21** (11), 3189–95.

4 Davison SN, Jhangri GS, Johnson JA (2006). Cross-sectional validity of a modified Edmonton symptom assessment system in dialysis patients: a simple assessment of symptom burden. *Kidney Int* **69** (9), 1621–5.

HRQL of dialysis patients

Dialysis treatment is promoted as a means of maintaining or improving a patient's quality of life and well-being. This inevitably results in patients electing to commence dialysis in the expectation that their lives will be significantly improved as a result of undergoing treatment.

However, studies based on Karnofsky, KDQOL, and SF-36, a patient's self-assessment quality of life health survey questionnaire, would indicate that the physical quality of life of both HD and PD patients is substantially impaired in comparison to the general population. Research suggests that HD patients experience lower levels of quality of life than PD patients in relation to physical functioning, role functioning, emotional and mental health, and pain, though such observations need to be adjusted for the lower comorbidity burden and younger average age of patients on PD. Comorbidities, low haemoglobin, and low residual renal function are all contributing factors to a poorer quality of life, as can be living alone with little or no support locally.

HRQL for PD patients

PD patients cite:
- feeling bloated;
- itching;
- feeling cold;
- lacking concentration;
- fatigue and difficulty mobilizing.

They also complain of:
- fear of infection;
- fear of having to convert to HD;
- anxiety about sexual intimacy;
- negative impact on sporting activities;
- negative impact on social life due to PD regime;
- feeling socially isolated;
- a lack of contact from the PD community team.

However, PD patients:
- usually find it easier to book holidays and short breaks as their dialysis fluid can be delivered to their holiday address or—if they are holidaying in the UK—they can often take their supplies with them;
- feel more in control of their lives and value their independence.

HRQL for HD patients

Some HD patients cite:
- ongoing fatigue;
- reduced physical activity and stamina;
- sleep disturbance;
- restless legs;
- leg cramps;
- itching;
- feeling cold;
- dizziness;

- headaches;
- nausea and vomiting;
- poor concentration;
- access problems;
- anxiety, panic attacks, and depression;
- erectile dysfunction.

They also cite feeling frustrated when trying to:
- arrange holidays or spontaneous short breaks;
- negotiate more flexible dialysis slots;
- avoid delays in being put on a machine;
- avoid unacceptable waiting times for hospital transport;
- maintain their role in the family.

HRQL for both HD and PD patients

For the great majority of people there is the hope of a transplant and continued disappointment as the wait continues.

It is perhaps not surprising to learn that, for some patients, the rigours of dialysis are barely tolerable. They struggle to integrate it into their lives and complain that having treatment has not in any way enhanced their quality of life.

Loss of control

Frequently mentioned in quality of life questionnaires is personal loss of control over one's own life and facing an uncertain future—a concern that is also shared by partners and family members.

'I am finding this whole thing so difficult and had I known it was going to be like this, I don't think I would have elected to have dialysis. I have to get up at an unearthly hour to be ready for transport. I invariably feel quite nauseated on the journey to the unit. I have to wait for up to an hour to be put on the machine and am then told off for having put on too much weight. Then I have to hang around waiting for transport to take me home by which time I am so tired I just flop into bed. What life is that? And the non-dialysis days are not much better as I still lack energy and 'get up and go'. It's not much fun for me and I know my family is suffering too. I feel such a burden—my husband has to do everything for me and, although he doesn't complain, he looks worn out. If I had known it was going to be like this, I would never have started it'

Expectations

It can be seen that some patients feel short-changed—that their expectations have not been met and that life on dialysis is not living. For other patients, the euphoria of being thrown a life-line can turn to despondency and despair as they recognize that their hopes of an enhanced quality of life were unrealistic. This is particularly so with patients whose underlying systemic disease was responsible for causing the ongoing progression of renal failure.

> Joanna was such a patient. She had cystic fibrosis and was diabetic, but a successful heart/lung transplant some 15 years previously had transformed her life. She had married and was able to hold down a fulltime job until her heart/lung anti-rejection drugs caused her kidneys to fail. She was also diagnosed with vasculitis and, as the disease progressed; she was readmitted to hospital where she underwent surgery to amputate first several of her fingers and then 2 weeks later above-knee amputations were performed. From being a totally independent and fully functioning person, in the space of just 8 weeks she became reliant upon nursing staff and family for her most basic needs. 'I can't even pick my own nose' she jokingly said but as the weeks passed, she became more and more dependent and despairing, saying 'Can you imagine what it's like having to ask a male nurse to wipe and wash your bottom?'

> 'There is nothing so useless as doing efficiently that which should not be done at all.'
>
> Peter Drucker

Whilst dialysis supports life, it doesn't necessarily improve quality of life and current research would indicate that the majority of dialysis-dependent patients rate HRQL as being less than 'good' as deteriorating health impacts on the amount of time they can spend at work and on other activities—to say nothing of the impact it has on family life.

Factors affecting quality of life

Fluctuating health and the rigours of dialysis impact on a patient's ability to be fully functioning.

Younger patients' complaints

- Being dialysis dependent sets them apart from their peers and accentuates 'difference'.
- Access surgery is 'mutilating' and affects perceptions of body image, which can deter patients from establishing meaningful relationships or initiating sexual activity.
- Fluid and dietary restrictions are difficult to reconcile with lifestyle and younger patients often find it easier to withdraw and isolate themselves from their peer group rather than risk participating and being labelled 'different'.
- Sometimes a desire to be socially included results in younger patients taking negative risks such as drug or alcohol abuse, disregarding dietary and fluid restrictions, or not attending for dialysis sessions.
- Parental involvement increases at a time when healthy separation should be occurring. This can lead to resentment, recriminations, and difficult family dynamics.

Older patients' complaints

They may be experiencing difficulty in:
- establishing and/or maintaining their role within the family;
- securing and/or sustaining employment;
- meeting existing financial commitments;
- fully participating in family activities, social events, and holidays;
- remaining sexually active;
- managing family dynamics and interpersonal relationships when all energy is invested in just trying to integrate dialysis into an existing daily routine.

They may find that they are more dependent upon family members.

General factors

Self-perception, self-worth, and self-esteem can be adversely affected by being dialysis-dependent, which can lead to relationship difficulties and in some cases relationship breakdown as the pressure of adjusting to dialysis becomes too difficult to manage. It can be a time when patients complain of feeling unsupported and not understood by their partners, carers, or indeed their physicians, and it is not uncommon for patients at this stage of their renal journey to consider withdrawal of treatment.

Conclusions

Conclusions

The impact of RRT will vary from modality used and from patient to patient. What is essential, however, is not to forget the importance of quality of life in assessing someone who is receiving dialysis and always to seek to see if there are ways it can be improved. Some factors such as transport, cited above, could be improved with better use of resources; others, particularly those that relate to comorbid conditions or complications of renal disease, may be irreversible. It is then important to strive to alleviate symptoms and provide all possible social, psychological, and spiritual support. This, the philosophy of palliative care, underpins the kind of care that we should endeavour to provide for these patients and their families and can be practised by any and all healthcare professionals, whatever the setting.

Further Reading

Further reading

Wight JP, Edwards L, Brazier J, *et al.* (1998). The SF36 as an outcome measure for end stage renal failure. *Qual Health Care* **7** (4), 209–21.

Maxwell P, Fitzpatrick R (1998). End-stage renal failure and assessment of health related quality of life. *Qual Health Care* **7**, 182.

Bakewell AB, Higgins RM, Edmunds ME (2002). Quality of life in PD patients—decline over time and association with clinical outcomes. *Kidney Int* **61**, 239–48.

The management of pain

Introduction

'Even thinking about pain is like tapping at a high voltage wire with the back of your finger to see if it's live.'

Christopher Wilson-Gleave

The growing number of patients on renal replacement therapy or conservative management of ESRD, many of whom have multiple comorbidities, means that there are many patients living with the consequences of their disease, one of which is an incidence of pain similar to that of cancer patients with metastatic disease. It is imperative that this is recognized by those caring for them and that pain is assessed and managed aggressively to improve quality of life. Management is made more difficult by the renal disease.

Incidence of pain

Studies indicate that between 50% and 67% of patients on dialysis experience significant pain.[1,2]

- Pain is moderate or severe for up to a half of those with pain.
- Significant numbers of patients are on no analgesia despite pain.
- Where the pain management index has been measured it indicates inadequate pain relief for three-quarters of patients.
- The mean duration of dialysis-related pain is 24 months:
  - it occurs more often than once a week;
  - the mean duration is 2h.
- The mean duration of pain not associated with the dialysis procedure is also 24 months.
- Some studies report an association between incidence of pain and length of time on dialysis.
- The mean pain score for both dialysis and non-dialysis pains shows that moderate to severe pain is experienced for both types.
- There is an association between pain and depression in ESRD.

Impact of pain

Using the Brief Pain Inventory scoring system to show how pain impacts on activities of every day reveals that it significantly affects:

- general activity;
- normal work;
- enjoyment of life;
- other aspects of life, such as walking ability, mood, and sleep, also but to a slightly lesser extent.

Causes of pain

The causes of pain in the ESRD population can be divided into categories. In some instances this will help the clinician determine the best management strategy.

Concurrent comorbidity

This is the most common cause of pain in this population.
- Diabetic neuropathy.
- Peripheral vascular disease.
- Chest pain.
- Arthritis.
- Decubitus ulcers.

Primary renal disease

A group of less common causes of pain, but may be a considerable challenge to relieve.
- Adult polycystic kidney disease (APKD):
  - pain from bleeding into or rupture of renal cysts;
  - pain from liver distension from liver cysts;
  - pain from infected liver cysts;
  - back pain from lumbar lordosis caused by longstanding abdominal distension from enlarged liver.
- Renal calculi.

Complications of renal failure

Some of these are the consequence of longevity achieved through successful renal replacement therapy. Although it may not always be possible to distinguish the precise cause of bone and joint pains, many of which are caused by comorbid arthritis, musculoskeletal pain from whatever cause constitutes the commonest single type of pain. This is important because it can also be a difficult group to treat as pain is often movement-related (see pp. 88 and 108).
- Renal osteodystrophy.
- Gout and other crystal arthropathies.
- Dialysis amyloid arthropathy.
- Calciphylaxis.

Infection
- Septic arthritis.
- Discitis with epidural abscess formation.
- Peritonitis in PD patients.

Dialysis-related pain
- 'Steal syndrome' from arteriovenous fistulas.
- Cramp.
- Headaches.
- Abdominal pain in PD patients.

References

1 Davison SN (2002). Pain in haemodialysis patients: prevalence, etiology, severity and analgesic use. *J Am Soc Nephrol* **42** (6), 1239–47.
2 Cornish C. (2005). A survey of pain in haemodialysis patients: prevalence, characteristics, management and impact. MSc dissertation.

Types of pain

For the purpose of management it is helpful to categorize pain into:

- nociceptive;
- neuropathic;
- mixed nociceptive and neuropathic;
- incident- or movement-related;
- other specific pains, e.g. colic, which may be of renal or gut origin.

Nociceptive pain or the pain due to tissue damage is usually responsive to opioid analgesia; the strength of analgesia needed will depend on the severity of the pain.

Neuropathic pain usually has some opioid sensitivity but the doses required to relieve pain may cause unacceptable side-effects. Adjuvant analgesics (discussed below; see p. 106) are therefore usually used with non-opioid and opioid analgesia. Many of the pains seen in ESRD are a mixture of both types, e.g. the pain of peripheral ischaemia. These therefore need a combination of opioid and adjuvant.

Incident- or movement-related pain often that caused by bone or joint damage, is more difficult to manage than most other pains. This is because pain is absent at rest when no or minimal analgesia is needed, but becomes very severe on movement requiring high levels of analgesia. This could lead to unacceptable side-effects, particularly sleepiness, if given at times when the patient has no pain.

Other specific causes It is important to diagnose other specific causes of pain, as there may be specific remedies to relieve them.

Assessment of pain

- Pain is what the patient says it is
- It can be affected by mood and the meaning of the pain

'It seems to me that pain in itself, though a pretty nasty piece of work, wouldn't have half the street cred if it wasn't like all bullies joined at the hip with that cringing lickspittle, fear'

Christopher Wilson-Gleave

Assessment of pain prior to initiation of management not only helps by determining, if possible, the cause of the pain, but also establishes a relationship with the patient. This relationship contributes to pain management through an ongoing partnership between physician or nurse and the patient. Pain relief is often not achieved at the first intervention but by initiating a plan of management, monitoring it, and adjusting it according to its effect on the patient. This ongoing commitment by the clinician to assess, reassess, and adjust gives the patient confidence that in itself will contribute to pain relief.

Areas covered by a pain assessment

- Site of pain.
- Duration of pain including whether it is:
  - constant;
  - intermittent;
  - day or night and whether it disturbs sleep.
- Provoking factors.
- Relieving factors.
- Radiation of pain.
- Intensity could be recorded as:
  - 'none', 'mild', 'moderate', or 'severe'; or
  - using a numerical rating scale 0–10 where 0 = no pain and 10 = pain as unbearable as you can imagine.
- Nature of pain, e.g. burning, stabbing.
- Presence of abnormal sensation.
- Mood (to exclude depression).
- Meaning of the pain to the individual.

Assessment tools

Formal assessment tools include the Brief Pain Inventory and McGill Pain Questionnaire both of which are validated for cancer patients but not for patients with ESRD. A modified version of the Edmonton Symptom Assessment System which includes pain has been validated in a group of dialysis patients.[1]

Figure 6.1 gives an example of an assessment system.

S   Site of pain: Where? Any radiation? Numbness where pain felt? Pattern of joint/muscle involvement?

O   Onset: When did it start? How did it start? What started it? Change over time? History or injury?

C   Character of pain: Type of pain — burning, shooting, stabbing, dull etc.

R   Radiation: Does the pain go anywhere else?

A   Associated feature

T   Timing/pattern: Is it worse at any time of day? Is it associated with any particular activities?

E   Exacerbating and relieving factors

S   Severity: Record especially if the pain is chronic and you want to measure change over time, consider a patient diary. Ask about:
- Pain intensity e.g. none—mild—moderate—severe; rank on a 1–10 scale.
- Record interference with sleep or usual activities.
- Pain relief e.g. none—slight—moderate—good—complete.

Fig. 6.1 Example of assessment system. (Taken with permission from O'Reilly K, Watson M (2007). *Pain and palliation*, Oxford General Practice Library. Oxford University Press, Oxford.)

References

1 Davison SN, Jhangri GS, Johnson JA (2006). Cross-sectional validity of a modified Edmonton symptom assessment system in dialysis patients: a simple assessment of symptom burden. *Kidney Int* **69**, 1621–5.

What hinders pain management?

Clinical factors

A combination of clinician and patient factors contribute to poor pain recognition and management in this group of patients. Some of these are listed below.

Clinician factors

- Lack of recognition of the problem and therefore failure to assess in the clinic.
- If pain reported, uncertainty as to how to manage it because of lack of training in pain management.
- Failure to monitor effect of treatment and therefore adjust according to response.
- Fear of causing toxicity from opioids.
- Fear of using strong opioids for non-cancer pain.
- Complex pain management because more than one cause of pain.

Patient factors

- Underreporting of pain in the clinic.
- Cause of pain not directly due to kidney function and therefore not seen as the role of the nephrologist to help it.
- Analgesia not taken for fear of side-effects.
- Analgesia stopped because of side-effects but without request for review.
- Unfounded fear of addiction.
- Unfounded fear of tolerance and loss of effectiveness in the future 'when stronger pain killers might be needed'.
- Delaying amputation leading to a longer period with limb ischaemia pain.

Drug handling in renal failure

Many drugs and their metabolites are excreted by the kidney through glomerular filtration, which, when reduced significantly, affects the clearance of those drugs and their metabolites. Where metabolites are active and retained as is the case for morphine, the likelihood of toxicity is high. Other factors also contribute to difficulty in prescribing analgesia effectively.

- Bioavailability varies more in patients with uraemia than in patients with normal renal function.
- Distribution:
  - increased in oedematous states;
  - decreased in dehydration and muscle wasting;
  - reduced plasma protein binding (especially acidic drugs, e.g. phenytoin) may lead to increased toxicity from greater availability of free drug.
- Metabolism:
  - in the liver is affected by high levels of urea; some metabolisms such as hydrolysis are slowed and others such as glucuronidation are not affected.

- Renal excretion (falls as GFR declines):
  - dependent on molecular size and protein binding of drug.
- Pharmacokinetics:
  - usually worked out by plasma drug/metabolite concentrations after one-off dose modelling;
  - application of this model to chronic dosing is limited;
  - guidelines for dose adjustments in handbooks can therefore only be regarded as useful approximations, and often conflict.
- Dialysis losses:
  - difficult to predict as many factors affect removal not just molecular size.

Further reading

Vidal L, Shavit M, Fraser A, et al. (2005). Systematic comparison of four sources of drug information regarding adjustment of dose for renal function. Br Med J **331**, 263–6.

Principles of management: the WHO analgesic ladder

Use of the WHO analgesic ladder (Fig. 6.2) to manage pain caused by cancer is recommended worldwide. Where pain is constant, as for many ESRD pains, a similar method of pain control can be used with modifications to take account of the effect of poor renal function. This method of working has been supported by a recent study looking at the efficacy of the WHO analgesic ladder in ESRD patients.[1]

The principles are as follows.
- By mouth—where the patient can swallow and absorb.
- By the clock—if pain constant, medication must be given regularly.
- By the ladder.
- With as needed, prn, medication if pain breaks through.
- For the individual.
- Attention to detail:
  - frequent assessment for efficacy and toxicity;
  - dose adjustments according to assessment;
  - aggressive management of side-effects.

Initial analgesia is selected according to the intensity of pain. When a VAS (visual analogue scale) of 0–10 is used, the following convention may be followed.
- Mild pain, scores 1–4:
  - step 1 on the WHO analgesic ladder.
- Moderate pain, scores 5–6:
  - step 2 on the WHO analgesic ladder.
- Severe pain, scores 7–10:
  - step 3 on the WHO analgesic ladder.

At all stages appropriate adjuvant treatment can be added. If pain is not adequately controlled move up the ladder or, if already on step 3, the strong opioid is titrated upwards to pain relief.

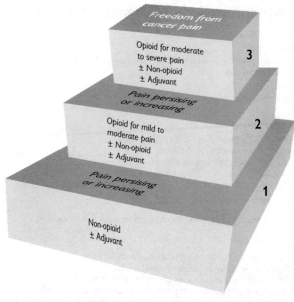

Fig. 6.2 The WHO analgesic ladder.

Reference

1 Barakzoy AS, Moss, AH (2006). Efficacy of the World Health Organization analgesic ladder to treat pain in end-stage renal disease. *J Am Soc Nephrol* **17** (11), 3198–203.

WHO analgesic ladder: steps 1 and 2

Step 1: non-opioids ± adjuvants

Paracetamol

Metabolized by the liver; metabolites do accumulate but accepted to be safe at normal doses.

Recommended: Paracetamol 1g qds

NSAIDs
- Should be avoided if residual renal function.
- Increase in non-renal side-effects.
- May be used in patients on dialysis.
  - Caution needed in PD patients with residual renal function.
- May be considered at end of life if best way of relieving pain.

± Adjuvants as indicated; see p. 106.

Step 2: opioids for mild to moderate pain + non-opioid ± adjuvants

Codeine
- Metabolized to codeine-6 glucuronide and morphine.
- Significant increase in half-life in renal failure.
- Accumulation of metabolites can cause drowsiness and confusion.
- Idiosyncratic response with prolonged narcosis in some individuals.
- If used, use in separate preparation from paracetamol and at reduced dose with careful monitoring.

Dihydrocodeine
- Reports of CNS depression.
- Little information in renal failure—*avoid*.

Dextropropoxyphene
- Avoid—metabolites toxic and accumulate.

Tramadol
- Agonist at μ opioid receptor.
- Metabolized in liver to O-desmethyltramadol.
- 90% excreted by kidney.
- 30% unchanged.
- Dose reduction recommended in renal failure:
  - use normal release preparations;
  - patients on dialysis 50mg tds–qds;
  - patients not dialysing 50mg bd.
- Watch for recognized side-effects—confusion and sedation.

Recommended: Tramadol 50mg bd (no dialysis); 50mg up to qds (dialysis) + non-opioids + adjuvants as indicated (see p. 106)

WHO step 3: opioids for moderate–severe pain + non-opioid ± adjuvant

Morphine

- Metabolized to morphine 3 glucuronide (M3G) and morphine-6-glucuronide (M6G).
- M6G more potent analgesic than morphine.
- M3G and M6G accumulate in renal failure and are not removed on dialysis.
- M6G thought to be the cause of significant toxicity with sedation, confusion, and myoclonic jerks with chronic dosing.
- *Not recommended for chronic use in renal failure*.

Hydromorphone

- Synthetic μ agonist; when used orally 4–7× as potent as oral morphine.
- Metabolized to hydromorphone 3 glucuronide (H3G) and other metabolites.
- Hydromorphone does not accumulate in ESRD, nor is it removed appreciably by dialysis.
- H3G, accumulates in renal failure but is removed by dialysis. However it is neurotoxic if injected intraventricularly in rats.
  - Two cases are reported of severe toxicity in patients, both of whom went into acute renal failure while taking doses of 1003mg hydromorphone parenterally daily (> 5000mg morphine equivalent) and 144mg orally (720mg morphine equivalent), respectively.
  - However, a further report, which demonstrated a high H3G to hydromorphone ratio in a patient with an estimated GFR of 19mL/min, describes the patient's cognitive function as normal.

Retrospective review and personal practice suggest the following for dialysis patients.
- Hydromorphone 1.3mg 4–6 hourly plus 1.3mg as needed if pain breaks through; can safely be used to titrate if step 3 analgesia required providing:
  - normal release preparations are used;
  - the patient is monitored carefully;
  - the total daily dose kept low by using TD fentanyl when > 12mg/day needed.

- Personal practice is to substitute transdermal fentanyl 25mcg/h when more than 9 doses of hydromorphone 1.3mg used in 24h and pain continuous.
- Hydromorphone is continued for breakthrough pain, increasing the breakthrough dose in line with the total 24h opioid dose (Table 6.1).

Oxycodone

- A semi-synthetic μ agonist with similar profile to morphine.
- 90% of the drug is metabolized in the liver with active metabolites.

Table 6.1 To show likely dose of prn hydromorphone needed according to fentanyl patch strength*

Fentanyl patch strength (mcg/h)	24h fentanyl dose (mcg)	4-hourly prn oral hydro-morphone (mg)	24-hourly morphine equivalent (mg)[‡]	4-hourly prn morphine equivalent (mg)[‡]
12	300	[†]	[†]	[†]
25	600	1.3–2.6	Up to 135	Up to 20
50	1200	2.6–3.9	135–224	25–35
75	1800	5.2	225–314	40–50
100	2400	6.5–7.8	315–404	55–65
125	3000	9.1	405–494	70–80

* All conversions are approximate and clinical judgement should be used at all times, starting at the lower end of the dose range and titrating upwards if needed.
[†] No data available.
[‡] Fentanyl/morphine equivalent doses taken from Durogesic drug information.

- Single dose study shows prolongation of elimination of both oxycodone and its main metabolite noroxycodone in patients with renal failure prior to transplant.
- Some anecdotal evidence of sedation and CNS toxicity.

- Limited evidence for its use in low doses in chronic renal failure; therefore cannot recommend for long-term use.

Buprenorphine

- A partial μ agonist/κ antagonist; sublingually 30–60 times as potent as oral morphine.
- Metabolized to buprenorphine-3-glucuronide (B3G) and norbuprenorphine (NorB) in the liver. Both accumulate significantly in renal failure.
- B3G is inactive.
- NorB has minor analgesic activity and causes respiratory depression in rats.
- A study of low dose transdermal (TD) buprenorphine in 10 haemodialysis patients who could tolerate the drug did not show excessive levels of NorB after a week.

- There is a lack of evidence about longer term use in ESRD.
- TD preparations should not be used for titration (see TD fentanyl).

Fentanyl
- Potent synthetic μ agonist 50–100 x as potent as morphine.
- 1000 x as lipophilic as morphine and therefore suitable for TD administration.
- Available for injection (IV or SC) or as a TD preparation.
- Metabolized in the liver to norfentanyl, which is inactive; therefore accumulation not clinically important.
- < 10% excreted unchanged in the urine.
- Preferred opioid for SC infusion at end of life, except where doses > 600mcg/24h required as volume required too large for portable syringe driver. See Chapter 12, p. 244.
- Preferred opioid for titration using prn SC administration at end of life even if alfentanil is being given via syringe driver as it has a longer duration of action than alfentanil when given SC.

- TD fentanyl can be used for stable, continuous pain in ESRD once the patient's opioid requirement has been titrated with an immediate release preparation and patient shown to tolerate equivalent opioid dose to patch prescribed (see Table 6.1).
- Patient should continue to be closely monitored.

Important considerations when using TD fentanyl
- Not appropriate for uncontrolled pain.
- Effective analgesia not reached until 24h after patch applied.
- When starting the first patch continue normal release medications for first 12h and ensure patient knows further doses may be needed while the dose of fentanyl from the patch builds up in the blood.
- A normal release strong opioid such as hydromorphone must be available for breakthrough pain.
- Maximum analgesia may not be reached until 72h so patch dose should not be increased until time for patch change.
- A depot of fentanyl remains under the skin for 24h after patch removal.
  - If naloxone needed to reverse narcosis a 24h infusion may be needed.
  - If pain relieved by another means, such as a nerve block or palliative radiotherapy, important to remember potential for toxicity from prolonged fentanyl action.
  - Patients should be monitored closely. In theory it might be expected that the dose could gradually be reduced, though no evidence from practice.

Alfentanil
- A derivative of fentanyl.
- It is one-quarter to one-fifth as potent as fentanyl but approximately 10 x more potent than SC diamorphine or 15 x as potent as SC morphine.
- It is extensively metabolized in the liver with inactive metabolites.

- Useful for continuous SC infusions because of greater solubility than fentanyl.
- Short duration of action when given SC so not useful for titrating opioid against pain relief (use fentanyl).
- But useful for short episodes of predictable pain, e.g. procedure-related pain.
- Buccal or nasal alfentanil can also be used for procedure-related pain. A solution of 5mg/5mL is available with a metered dose of 0.14mg per activation (see p. 107).
  - This has the advantage to the patient of self-administration.

Methadone

- Synthetic opioid active at μ opioid receptor.
- Thought to have some activity as an NMDA receptor antagonist and therefore possible role in neuropathic pain.
- It is excreted mainly in the faeces, but also metabolism in the liver to inactive metabolites.
- In the anuric patient excretion is almost exclusively faecal.
- Methadone titration for pain control with normal renal function needs specialist experience because of its prolonged pharmacological action—up to 60h.

- Characteristics suggest it may be safe in patients with ESRD but only in the hands of those experienced in its use for pain control in patients with normal renal function.

Recommended: Hydromorphone titrated using a normal release preparation: 1.3mg capsule orally until > 9 doses/24h needed consistently. Then stop regular hydromorphone and use TD fentanyl 25mcg/h as background analgesia and continue titrating with normal release hydromorphone. See 'Summary', p. 102, and above. Close monitoring for toxicity required at all times

Parenteral opioids

- Preferred route subcutaneous.
- Preferred strong opioid for titrating and breakthrough pain: fentanyl.
  - Suggested doses 12.5–25mcg SC prn hourly (titrate to higher dose if needed).
  - For doses greater than 600mcg/24h use alfentanil.

For full details see Chapter 12, p. 231, and 'Summary', p. 102.

Summary: WHO analgesic ladder

General points
- Assess the patient's pain.
- Choose appropriate step.
- Give drug regularly plus prn for breakthrough pain or incident pain.
- Monitor for toxicity and efficacy.
- Adjust and move up a step or increase dose as needed.
- Remember psychological, social, and spiritual distress will impact on pain.

Step 1: non-opioid ± adjuvants Paracetamol 1g qds ± adjuvants including NSAIDs if safe and indicated.

Step 2: non-opioid + opioid for mild–moderate pain ± adjuvants
Paracetamol 1g qds + tramadol 50mg bd (no dialysis) to qds (dialysis) 9 adjuvants including NSAIDs if indicated and safe.

If using codeine, 30mg qds to a maximum 120mg/24h; prescribe separately from paracetamol.

Step 3: non-opioid + opioid for moderate–severe pain ± adjuvants

Patient able to swallow oral medication
Paracetamol 1g qds +

1 Hydromorphone 1.3mg 4–6 hourly regularly plus 1.3mg prn for breakthrough pain.
2 If pain not controlled, continuous, and 24h dose hydromorphone exceeds 12mg or > 9 doses of 1.3mg, substitute TD fentanyl 25mcg/h for regular hydromorphone. Continue with hydromorphone for breakthrough pain (see Table 6.1).
3 If further 'as needed' hydromorphone exceeds 12mg/24h increase dose of fentanyl patch by further 25mcg.
4 Continue to titrate upwards in similar manner if pain not controlled.

± adjuvants as indicated.

Patient unable to swallow oral medication For details see Chapter 12 (pp. 242–5) and Fig. 6.3.

Opioid naïve
1 Fentanyl 12.5–25mcg SC prn up to hourly available whether pain present or not.
2 If > 2–3 prn doses needed in 24h set up SC syringe driver.
3 Dose in syringe driver depends on previous requirements, but suitable starting dose is 100–250mcg/24h.
4 Plus SC fentanyl 12.5–25mcg prn hourly.

Already on strong opioids For details see Chapter 12 (pp. 242–5), Table 6.1 (p. 99), and Fig. 6.3.
1 Convert to dose equivalent SC fentanyl in a syringe driver.
2 If > 600mcg fentanyl required, use alfentanil.
3 Increase dose according to previous day's prn doses and add to the regular dose (do not include doses used for specific movement/incident-related pain, e.g. dressing change or washing).
4 Plus prn SC fentanyl; approximately one-tenth of the 24h fentanyl dose, prn hourly.

The WHO analgesic ladder can be used in renal patients *drug and dose modification suggested* for use in renal failure

Note: this is a guide and analgesia should always be tailored for the individual patient.

At end of life analgesia should always be prescribed by an appropriate route in anticipation of symptoms; the preferred parenteral route is subcutaneous

Parenteral drugs prescribed in anticipation of pain:

Fentanyl 12.5–25 micrograms prn hourly: can be used to titrate or for painful procedures such as dressing change If patient already on TD fentanyl or by syringe driver: the prn dose is approx 1/10th the 24 hour dose

Starting syringe driver (SD) doses for the opioid-naive: fentanyl 100–150 micrograms/24 hours

Step 3: Oral:

Hydromorphone HD/PD: 1.3mg 4–6 hourly + 1.3 mg prn; convert to **TD fentanyl** HD/PD: 12 or 25 microgram/hr q72h based on previous opioid dose if pain continous

Subcutaneous: fentanyl see box above

Alfentanil use when SD contains > 600micrograms fentanyl/24 hours

Alfentanil is 1/4 as potent as fentanyl; prn doses are very short lasting ∴useful for incident pain, e.g. dressing change but not for titration.

Prn alfentanil dose is 1/10th the 24 hour dose

3. Opioid for moderate–severe pain
± non-opioid
± adjuvant

Step 2:

Tramadol:
HD/PD: 50 mg qds
Conservative pathway 50mg bd

Codeine
HD/PD:15–30mg qds

2. Opioid for mild–moderate pain
± non-opioid
± adjuvant

Adjuvants: can be used at all levels

Gabapentin PO
HD: loading 300mg
Maintenance 200–300mg post HD
PD: 300mg alternate days
Renal impairment: dependent on GFR

Amitriptyline PO
HD/PD: 10–25mg on the titrate gradually

NSAIDs:
Conservative pathway: AVOID
HD/PD: use low dose for short courses if necessary: consider gastric protection e.g. Ibuprofen 200mg tds
Diclofenac 25mg tds

Step 1:

Paracetamol PO/IV/PR 1g qds
± adjuvant

1. Non-opioid
± adjuvant

Increasing pain

Consult your local palliative care team for advice where pain difficult to control or for dose conversions

Fig. 6.3 Guidance on the use of analgesics in renal patients, including end of life care.

Managing opioid side-effects

Many side-effects from opioids are predictable. This should be explained and appropriate measures taken. Others are less predictable but clinicians should assess for unwanted effects and attempt to alleviate them. Many side-effects mimic the symptoms from uraemia and it can be difficult to distinguish them; opioids are frequently stopped when confusion, sedation, or agitation occurs. When the clinical situation has been assessed it is important not to leave the patient without adequate analgesia, and to retitrate using normal release oral preparations of hydromorphone or SC fentanyl.

If a patient who was on a stable dose of analgesia without toxicity becomes toxic it is likely there has been a change in the clinical situation that needs considering and managing such as:

- infection;
- dehydration;
- other electrolyte disturbance;
- worsening of poor renal function;
- myocardial infarction.

Side-effects

- Nausea and vomiting:
    - occur in approximately a quarter of patients;
    - wear off after 10–14 days;
    - make antiemetic available when starting opioids (see Chapter 7, pp. 128–31).
- Constipation:
    - nearly universal;
    - provide all patients with laxatives (see Chapter 7, pp. 132–3).

Central nervous system effects

- Drowsiness:
    - more common when first starting opioid or increasing the dose;
    - may reduce after 72h;
    - if continues consider alternative opioid, or alternative means of pain control.
- Confusion:
    - occurrence as for drowsiness;
    - more likely with morphine (see p. 98);
    - exclude correctable associations (see above);
    - reduce dose;
    - consider alternative opioid or means of pain relief.
- Myoclonic jerks:
    - most commonly caused by morphine;
    - stop morphine;
    - substitute alternative; see p. 98.
- Respiratory depression is **not** a problem if:
    - dose of opioids titrated upwards against pain because patients become tolerant to the respiratory depressant effect;
    - short-acting preparations are used for titration;

- dose titration takes place prior to placement of a fentanyl patch;
- pain is suddenly relieved by a procedure such as nerve block and systemic analgesia is stopped and retitrated.
- Respiratory depression *can* occur however:
  - when clinical situation changes;
  - pain is reduced but analgesia is not;
  - if patient not carefully monitored.

Adjuvant analgesia

Adjuvant drugs, whose prime indication may not be pain, are used in specific clinical situations to relieve pain and are often more effective than opioids in those situations and therefore less likely to cause toxicity. Many need modification to their doses in renal failure. See Chapter 15.

Pain syndromes

Neuropathic pain Many pains in ESRD are neuropathic in nature or mixed nociceptive and neuropathic. These usually need a combination of opioid and adjuvant for optimal effect.

- Antidepressants:
  - good evidence for tricyclic antidepressants;
  - number needed to treat (NNT) = 3;
  - number needed to harm (NNH) = 22;
  - side-effects, particularly dry mouth and sedation, usually limit dose achievable;
  - titrate slowly from very low doses, i.e. start amitryptyline at 10mg nocte.
- Anticonvulsants:
  - NNT = 2.9;
  - NNH = 8;
  - gabapentin—doses must be reduced in renal failure (see Fig. 6.3);
  - clonazepam—useful as easy to titrate, rapid response (see Chapter 12, pp. 231–2, 244);
  - carbamazepine—may be difficult to use because of drug interactions and patients usually on multidrug regimens.
- Topical measures: see below.

Colic—bowel obstruction

- Hyoscine butylbromide
  - give parenterally 20mg SC prn 2 hourly; or
  - in syringe driver: dose required varies from 80 to 120mg/24h SC.

Renal colic

- NSAIDs first choice unless absolute contraindication.
- Hysocine butylbromide 2nd choice.
- May need opioids: first choice is SC fentanyl.

Muscle spasm

- Benzodiazepines:
  - diazepam if able to swallow;
  - midazolam at end of life;
  - clonazepam single night-time dose.
- Baclofen.

Topical methods of analgesia

Opioids

Opioids may be effective topically where the skin is broken and there is inflammation as opioid receptors migrate to areas of inflammation. Most experience relates to morphine in a hydrogel such as Intrasite gel, though other opioids such as fentanyl and diamorphine have been used. As the effect is local and relatively low doses are used it is thought that there is little effect from systemic absorption.

- Indications:
  - ischaemic leg ulcer that is painful between dressing changes;
  - decubitus ulcer for which treatment is palliative and healing not expected.
- Possible prescription:
  - morphine (for injection) 10mg in Intrasite gel applied to the ulcer daily.

Capsaicin cream

Capsaicin is a chilli alkaloid that depletes substance P. There is evidence for benefit when it is used for postherpetic neuralgia, diabetic neuropathy, and osteoarthritis though a significant proportion of people will not tolerate it as it causes burning prior to relief. Possible uses:

- localized areas of neuropathic pain from diabetic neuropathy (NNT, 4);
- osteoarthritis (NNT, 3).

Topical NSAIDs These may be useful for localized joint pain, with non-ulcerated skin and when systemic NSAID is contraindicated (NNT, 3).

Buccal, nasal, or sublingual alfentanil

Reasonable bioavailability and good solubility mean that a sufficient dose of alfentanil can be given buccally to achieve short-term (15–20min) analgesia to cover painful procedures or planned painful activities. The provision of metered dosing delivering 0.14mL (0.14mg) per spray enables the patient to have control. The dose required will vary from patient to patient but it is reasonable to start with three sprays, which delivers a dose of 0.42mg, increasing the number of sprays if needed. Doses greater than 1.5mL are likely to be swallowed rather than absorbed buccally so are unlikely to be effective. This use of alfentanil is an off-label use of the drug and should be monitored.

KJ was a 72-year-old lady with myeloma. She developed a 9cm lytic lesion in her left iliac bone with bony expansion and destruction; there was an associated lesion in the left femur with cortical destruction. Her renal function was significantly impaired. While she waited for the benefit of the palliative radiotherapy that she received to the lesions, she was nursed in bed as all movement was excruciating. At rest in bed she was pain-free on her background analgesia. In order to mobilize on to the commode, she used three sprays of alfentanil, and was then able to move in relative comfort; she usually used a second dose of alfentanil prior to returning to her bed. After the radiotherapy treatment she returned home and continued to use the buccal alfentanil in decreasing frequency over the following month until there had been sufficient healing for movement to no longer be painful.

Episodic, movement-related, or incident pain

These terms describe pain that occurs despite regular analgesic medication. They can be divided into the following.

Spontaneous episodes of pain

- Usually neuropathic.
- May be short-lived but severe.
- Shooting or burning in nature.
- No precipitating factors.
- Consider neuropathic agent for pain relief.

Breakthrough pain occurring during dose titration

- Background analgesia inadequate.
- Occurs at end of dosing period indicating higher dose needed.
- Explain to patient and continue dose titration.
- Dose of breakthrough medication related to the 24h opioid taken:
  - for hydromorphone, morphine, and oxycodone: 1/6th 24h dose;
  - for fentanyl and alfentanil: 1/10th 24h dose titrating up to 1/6th if ineffective.

Movement-related or incident pain

- Patient pain-free at rest but severe pain on movement or dressing change.
- Gradually titrate background opioid to highest level tolerated by the patient.
- Use short-acting opioid prior to planned activity, e.g. dressing change. Choose drug and route depending on patient's condition and length of procedure:
  - oral hydromorphone: onset 30min, duration 4h;
  - SC fentanyl: onset 5–10min, duration 1–2h;
  - SC alfentanil: onset 3–5min, duration about 30–60min;
  - buccal/nasal/sublingual alfentanil: onset 5–10min, duration 20min.
- Entonox (inhaled nitrous oxide) may have a role for episodes of care in those who are not too frail.
- Look for local means of relieving pain, e.g. joint immobilization.
- Consider nerve blocks or anaesthetic procedure.

Chronic pain clinic referral and anaesthetic procedures

In some situations severe chronic pain management can be exceedingly difficult and the patient may be helped by referral to a chronic pain management team where they may benefit from management by their multidisciplinary pain team.

Anaesthetic procedures may be indicated in some of the following situations:

• severe neuropathic pain where spinal analgesia could be an option;
• incident pain, such as that from a fractured hip where patient not fit for surgery, for local anaesthetic block;
• sympathetically mediated pain;
• difficulty in achieving satisfactory pain control despite escalating analgesia or because of unacceptable toxicity when analgesia is achieved.

Referral to the palliative care team

Referral to the palliative care team

When pain is difficult to manage or there are other distressing symptoms or psychological or social issues, referral to your local palliative care team may give the opportunity for a holistic assessment and review with improvement in symptoms. The presence of severe pain when part of disease progression and patient deterioration often indicates that prognosis is reduced or short. It should therefore act as a trigger for referral to a palliative care service. This can occur even if prognosis is uncertain, as good symptom relief and support should improve quality of life. It may also enable discussions about future care to be started. See also Chapter 10.

Further reading

Dean M (2004). Opioids in renal failure and dialysis patients. *J Pain Symptom Manage* **28**, 497–504.

Ferro CJ, Chambers EJ, Davison SN (2004). Management of pain in renal failure. In *Supportive care for the renal patient* (ed. Chambers EJ, Germain M, Brown E), pp. 105–53. Oxford University Press, Oxford.

Kurella M, Bennett WM, Chertow GM (2003). Analgesia in patients with ESRD: a review of available evidence. *Am J Kid Dis* **42** (2) 217–28.

Murtagh FEM, Chai MO, Donohoe P, *et al.* (2007). The use of opioid analgesia in end-stage renal disease patients managed without dialysis: recommendations for practice. *J Pain Palliat Care Pharmacother* **21** (2) (accepted for publication).

Non-pain symptoms in end-stage renal disease

Introduction

Patients with end-stage renal disease are one of the most symptomatic groups of patients with chronic diseases. A systematic review of the prevalence of symptoms in patients undergoing dialysis revealed that fatigue/tiredness, pruritus, and constipation occur in more than half of dialysis patients and over 40% experience anorexia, pain, and sleep disturbance. An ongoing study of symptoms in the patient who has chosen the conservative pathway shows a broadly similar incidence of fatigue/tiredness, pruritus, anorexia, and sleep disturbance, but pain seems to be experienced by a greater proportion of patients.

Assessment in a busy clinic is time-consuming, but other members of the renal team could contribute, perhaps through the use of assessment tools such as the dialysis symptom index or the Edmonton symptom assessment system.

The high prevalence of symptoms in this group of patients is due to the combination of those from chronic uraemia, those from the other comorbid conditions, many of which are responsible for their renal disease, and those that are the result of renal replacement therapy (RRT). Pain in chronic dialysis patients is as common as for patients with metastatic cancer with 40–55% of patients suffering from moderate to severe pain. Of non-pain symptoms in dialysis patients:

- mean number of symptoms per patient = 9;[1,2]
- worst symptoms:
  - tiredness;
  - lack of well being;
  - poor appetite.

In patients on conservative management:
- Mean number of symptoms = 6.[3]

The overall effect of this symptom burden is reduced quality of life, which correlated with higher symptom burden in a group of dialysis patients with high comorbidity.

Causes of the common non-pain symptoms

These can be divided into:
- those directly related to uraemia;
- those related to the longevity achieved through renal failure management;
- those caused by comorbid conditions;
- those directly related to the dialysis procedure.

Important management considerations for all patients

Ensure:
- adequate dialysis;
- anaemia management;
- treatment of iron deficiency.

Table 7.1 Symptom burden in ESRD patients on dialysis and those managed conservatively

Symptom	Prevalence (%) in patients	
	On dialysis[3]	Treated conservatively (early; n = 472)[4]
Fatigue/weakness	71	70
Pruritus	55	55
Anorexia	49	49
Pain	47	62
Sleep disturbance	44	39
Anxiety	38	34
Dyspnoea	35	39
Nausea	33	27
Restless legs	30	28
Depression	27	28

References

1 Davison SS, Jhangri GS, Johnson JA (2006). Cross-sectional validity of a modified Edmonton symptom assessment system in dialysis patients: a simple assessment of symptom burden. *Kidney Int* **69** (9), 1621–5.

2 Weisbord SD, Fried LE, Arnold RM, et al. (2005). Prevalence, severity and importance of physical and emotional symptoms in chronic haemodialysis patients. *J Am Soc Nephrol* **16** (8), 2487–94.

3 Murtagh FEM, Addington-Hall J, Higginson IJ (2007). The prevalence of symptoms in end-stage renal disease: a systematic review. *Adv Chronic Kidney Dis* **14** (1): 82–89.

4 Unpublished data. Murtagh FEM, Murphy E, Watson S (2006). Symptoms in end-stage renal disease: an evaluation of symptoms in patients with end-stage renal disease managed conservatively at Guy's Hospital and King's College Hospital renal units. Internal report published 19th February 2006.

Pruritus and dry skin

Pruritus occurs in more than 50% of HD and PD patients, with about half of those patients rating it as moderate or severe. In a study of 1773 haemodialysis patients, 25% scored itch > 7 on a visual analogue scale (0–10).[1] This was confirmed by a more recent study showing 46% rating it moderate or severe.[2] It is a very unpleasant symptom associated with reduced quality of life.

Characteristics of pruritus in ESRD

- No relation with the type of dialysis, either HD or PD.
- Some studies report a relationship between the timing of the appearance of the symptom and receiving dialysis, but the reports conflict and the following have been reported:
  - increase in incidence while dialysing;
  - peak in the period preceding dialysis;
  - lowest incidence immediately following dialysis.
- However, it may occur all the time or be transient in nature.
- May be localized or generalized.
- Is often worse at night.
- Three-quarters of those who rate it severe experience sleep disturbance.
- Severe pruritus is more common in males, though itch overall may be more common in women.
- Skin appearance ranges from the normal to severe xerosis with or without secondary skin changes from repeated scratching.
- High levels of urea, calcium, and phosphate, and low levels of ferritin and albumin associated with increased incidence.
- Reduced incidence associated with low calcium levels.
- Exacerbating factors include: heat, rest, dry skin, and sweat.

Pathophysiology of pruritus in ESRD

The pathophysiology is complex and multifactorial. The relative importance of different aetiological factors will vary from patient to patient, so an individual assessment of likely key causes may help guide management plans. The perception of pruritus follows a normal sensation pathway from receptors in the skin, probably non-myelinated C fibres though no specific receptor has been identified, with transmission to the cortex. Likely mechanisms include the following.

- Dermal mast cell proliferation.
  - Associated with increased histamine, serotonin (though no clear relationship between levels and severity), and cytokines all released by mast cells.
- Possible interaction between mast cells and C fibres (i.e. a form of neuropathy).
  - This may be associated with abnormal pattern of cutaneous innervation.
- Other theories include:
  - secondary hyperparathyroidism;
  - possible low grade sensitivity to dialysis products.

General management
For nearly all ESRD-related non-pain symptoms an important aspect of their management includes optimal management of the following:
- dialysis prescription;
- nutritional status;
- anaemia;
- calcium and phosphate product.

Management strategies for pruritus
A multitude of diverse therapies has been tried for uraemic pruritus. Evidence for some is conflicting. This is probably because studies have been small and the condition is multifactorial. The effectiveness of treatment will depend on aetiology. Where this is known, appropriately directed therapy can be instituted.

General measures
- Exacerbating factors, which will vary for individuals, such as hot baths and alcohol should be avoided.
- Maintenance of skin moisture by means of:
  - emollients with high water content;
  - avoiding soap;
  - use of emulsifying ointments in bath.
- Light clothing. Non-synthetic may be better than some synthetics.
- Discourage scratching—short nails, gloves at night.
- Showers, both hot and cold, help some individuals.
- Improve sleep.

Topical treatments
- Capsaicin cream, has been shown to be helpful for some patients:
  - likely to be most useful in localized itching;
  - some patients cannot tolerate it because of the burning it causes.
- Tacrolimus ointment. A prospective study of 27 patients showed a significant reduction in pruritus score with no systemic effects. However, time to response is not recorded and 4 patients withdrew.
- There is no evidence for the use of topical steroids and their potential side-effects weaken any argument for using them.

Specific measures
The following have been shown to be effective for some patients. Treatment decisions will be taken on an individual patient basis depending on circumstances, burden of treatment, its requirement for monitoring (e.g. thalidomide), or potential for adverse effects. Time to efficacy has not been reported for all treatments and this will be a crucial for patients near the end of their life.
- Ultraviolet B phototherapy. Consistent evidence for effectiveness offset in this population by burden of treatment.
- Antihistamines. Little evidence but continue to be used by patients. It is simple to use them and to monitor benefit and adverse effects.

- Gabapentin. One study of 25 patients using thrice weekly gabapentin after dialysis showed a significant reduction in pruritus score.
  - In patients with an estimated GFR < 15 the suggested dose might be 300mg alternate days, monitoring carefully for toxicity.
- Thalidomide. Cross-over randomized, placebo-controlled trial of 29 patients: half the patents had significant reduction in pruritus; none responded to placebo. Prescription, controlled handling, and sedative side-effects may make this inappropriate at end of life.

Initial reports of benefit from ondansetron, naltrexone, and erythropoietin have not been confirmed and larger studies are needed to determine their place in the management of itch. Where vomiting, which is not otherwise controlled, is also a problem, ondansetron might be considered but its use is offset by headache and constipation and other antiemetics may be more effective.

References

1 Narita I, Alchi B, Omori K, *et al.* (2006). Etiology and prognostic significance of severe uremic pruritus in chronic hemodialysis patients. *Kidney Int* **69** (9), 1626–322.
2 Davison SN, Jhangri GS, Johnson JA. (2006) Cross-sectional validity of a modified Edmonton symptom assessment system in dialysis patients. A simple assessment of symptom burden. *Kidney Int* **69** (9) 1621–625.

Fatigue, daytime somnolence, and weakness

This common symptom complex is experienced by:
- over two-thirds of patients before the onset of dialysis;
- a similar proportion after starting RRT;
- one-third of conservatively managed patients.

Poor sleep, discussed below, is associated with daytime somnolence and reduced quality of life.
- 45% of 507 dialysis patients rated drowsiness as moderate or severe.
- Muscle weakness itself will contribute to fatigue and reduced mobility and activity.
- This may lead to further reduction in activity and hence further muscle weakness with the potential for a spiral downwards of function if not actively managed.

There is some evidence that the level of impairment correlates with the level of renal impairment and that, by the time patients are on RRT, overall their function is at a lower level than that of pre-dialysis patients.

Important factors contributing to the development of lethargy
- Inadequate dialysis.
- Uraemia.
- Anaemia:
  - iron deficiency;
  - low erythropoietin levels.
- Biochemical abnormalities, particularly hyper- or hypokalaemia, hypomagnesaemia, hyper- or hypocalcaemia, hyponatraemia, and hypophosphataemia.
- Poor nutritional state.
- Poor quality sleep.
- Depression.
- Renal bone disorders leading to reduced activity because of pain.
- Pain.

Impact of fatigue and weakness
In the dialysis patient this symptom complex has a major impact on quality of life. Reduced levels of functioning will impair social activities and may prevent the ability to work or run the household; this has an ongoing effect that spreads beyond the patient to those close to them. Loss of role, such as bread winner or household manager, leads to loss of self-esteem with the potential for depression and psychological distress. As functioning decreases, the need for hospital transport to and from dialysis sessions with associated stress and frustration leads to further reduction in quality of life

By the time many patients with ESRD consider stopping dialysis their performance status is very low with increasing need for assistance with activities of daily living. This may be one of the factors that precipitates discussion about dialysis cessation. Function will worsen as a result of stopping and the need for considerable care can prevent patients dying in their place of choice, if such care is unavailable at short notice either at home or in a nursing home.

Fatigue, like pain in the ESRD patient, is associated with depression, itself difficult to diagnose in the presence of chronic physical disease with many similar symptoms.

Post-dialysis fatigue Some patients experience severe fatigue immediately post-dialysis. This may relate to rapid changes in fluid volume, an effect on BP, or depletion of specific substances during dialysis. There is an expectation among patients that they will feel better when dialysis starts; for the frail and elderly the reverse may happen and they may actually feel worse. These are important considerations when decisions are being made about whether or not to start dialysis. See also Chapters 9, 11, and 12.

Management
The management of fatigue and weakness will depend on the stage of the person's illness. What is appropriate when the prognosis is measured in months or years is unlikely to be appropriate in the last weeks and days of someone's life.

General non-drug measures
Will include optimizing dialysis (if relevant), the medical management of the patient's other medical conditions, anaemia correction, and attention to patient's nutritional status as possible and appropriate.
- Physiotherapy and gentle rehabilitation programmes are associated with improved exercise tolerance and reduced fatigue, but may not be appropriate.
- As disease advances, social care to optimize support for everyday living and later nursing care are likely to be needed by many patients.
- Ensuring a good night's sleep if possible.
- Acupressure. Two studies from Taiwan suggest acupressure is helpful in reducing the severity of fatigue, though this may not either be available or applicable to patients at the end of life.

Specific and drug measures
- Optimal anaemia management should continue till the last few days of life. There is good evidence that treating anaemia in dialysis patients reduces fatigue.
  - Erythropoietin;
  - Iron therapy. See Chapter 3 (p. 40).
- Screen for and treat depression if present.

Anorexia and weight loss

Clinical protein/energy malnutrition is common; dialysis patients require twice the protein of a non-dialysing patient. Malnutrition is associated with raised inflammatory markers and likely to have a similar aetiology to cancer and cardiac cachexia. It is strongly associated with increased morbidity and mortality.

About one-half of patients on dialysis and a similar proportion of those managed conservatively without dialysis experience significant anorexia. It is multifactorial and the following may all have a bearing in some patients.

- Chronic nausea.
- Dry mouth, with or without superimposed mouth infections.
- Altered taste.
- Delayed gastric emptying from diabetic neuropathy, or medication such as opioids.
- Restricted ESRD diet limiting food options leading to reduced intake.
- Lower bowel abnormalities, such as constipation, diabetic enteropathy, or ischaemic bowel symptoms.
- Fatigue exhausting the patient so too tired to eat food they have prepared.
- Social isolation. Eating alone can led to reduced intake.
- Depression.
- Under dialysis.
- Uraemia.
- Hypokalaemia resulting from poor nutrition.
- Abdominal discomfort and swelling from PD.

Management

All the conditions described above that can be reversed or partially reversed should be attended to. The advice of a renal dietician should be sought. The goals of this advice will change when renal replacement therapy is discontinued and the aim is comfort. The liberalization of diet that ensues may be helpful to the patient. Some aspects of the attention to detail that follows may be helpful to patients.

- Treat mouth infections, particularly thrush.
- Review drugs for those that cause dry mouth to see if any can be discontinued.
- Manage dry mouth actively where it is a problem. See p. 126.
- Trial of metoclopramide (in the absence of nausea or vomiting it may help by increasing the rate of gastric emptying and reducing early satiety). NB. Most effective if taken 20–30min before meals.
- Tempt the patient with small, well presented meals that they have chosen or are known to like.
- Unless the patient wishes to eat alone, eating in company is associated with a greater input.
- Reduce fatigue during eating by thoughtful presentation or help with eating.
- Treat depression.

Appetite stimulants

Steroids such as dexamethasone 2–4mg daily may temporarily increase appetite and sense of well-being, though there is no evidence for muscle weight gain.

- Effect is of short duration; defined course should be prescribed with a specific aim and with review of efficacy.
- Possible short-term ill effects such as fluid retention must be balanced against any potential gain.

Dry mouth and thirst

Both dry mouth and thirst are common accompaniments to end-stage renal disease and dialysis. Objective studies have shown a clear relationship between thirst and xerostomia as measured by salivary flow.

Most patients will have devised their own strategies for minimizing and alleviating this symptom with common sense strategies such as keeping out of the sun, limiting salt in food, and the avoidance of commercial drink outlets.

There are no good studies to guide management but some evidence for:
- chewing gum (small cross-over study);
- artificial saliva;
- pilocarpine (observational study).

Nausea

- Present for up to a third of dialysis patients.
- It is thought mainly to relate to uraemia: however:
  - it is likely the body develops a degree of tolerance to the emetic effect of urea and other toxins;
  - it is possible that nausea is more likely when there are sudden rises in urea.

Other relevant factors include the following.
- Fluid and electrolyte changes.
- Concurrent medication can contribute to nausea in two ways:
  - chemical stimulation, e.g. antibiotics, opioids;
  - delayed gastric emptying, e.g. amitryptyline, opioids.
- The presence of infection.
- Delayed gastric emptying from other causes such as diabetic enteropathy.
- Constipation.

Causes unrelated to ESRD must of course be looked for and treated appropriately. Vomiting is not commonly present unless there are other medical complications at the time.

Management of nausea and vomiting See Table 7.2.
Many of the general measures that apply to anorexia also apply here and can be used in conjunction with Table 7.2, which lists possible causes, suggested first-line drugs with as needed additional medication, and second-line drugs where available. It aims to help the tailoring of anti-emesis to the putative cause. These suggestions are largely empirically based as there is little evidence, though the underlying scheme is widely accepted in palliative care.

Principles of antiemetic prescribing
- Consider probable cause.
- Select appropriate antiemetic.
- If nausea or vomiting constant, prescribe medication regularly up to full dose.
- It may be necessary to prescribe additional medication as needed if nausea or vomiting break through the regular antiemetic.
- Review effect and reconsider cause or adequacy of route if ineffective.
- If unable to swallow or vomiting oral antiemetics or at end of life,
  - use SC route and, if symptoms constant, use syringe driver.
    See also Chapter 12, pp. 238, 245.

Questions to ask if treatment fails
- Is antiemetic appropriate to cause?
- If oral administration:
  - is drug being taken?
  - is drug lost through vomiting?
  - is drug being absorbed?
- Is drug at maximum safe dose?

When those factors corrected for, consider the following

- Adding 2nd-line drug; *or*
- changing to 2nd-line or broad spectrum antiemetic (Table 7.2); *or*
- changing to 24h SC administration (this can be a temporary solution to break the cycle of vomiting and if patient well enough return to the oral route).

If nausea intractable and all treatment only partially effective, the addition of dexamethasone at doses of 2–6mg per day may enhance the effect of other antiemetics. Whether this is due to a reduction in the blood–brain barrier or other undefined mechanism is not known. This can be given as an od SC injection.

Table 7.2 Antiemetics in ESRD

Site or mode of action Neurotransmitter(s)	Direct stimulants	1st-line	Use in ESRD	prn drug	2nd-line
Chemoreceptor trigger zone (CTZ) D2, 5HT$_3$	Chemicals: uraemia, drugs	Haloperidol 0.5–1.5mg PO/SC od or tds	No dose reduction necessary	Haloperidol 0.5mg up to 5mg/24h	Levomepromazine 6mg PO or 5mg SC prn up to 8-hourly
Vomiting centre stimulated indirectly by CTZ, higher centres, & vestibular afferents H$_1$, 5HT$_2$, Ach$_m$	Autonomic afferents: abdomen, thorax	Cyclizine 50mg 8-hourly	No dose reduction, but increases dry mouth. Avoid in acute coronary events	Levomepromazine 5mg PO/SC prn up to 8-hourly	Levomepromazine 6mg PO or 5mg SC prn up to 8-hourly
Cerebral cortex	Fear, anxiety, pain	Benzodiazepine: lorazepam 1mg SL, diazepam 2mg	Caution with repeated doses: metabolite accumulation	Additional 1st-line drug, but accumulation with increasing doses	Levomepromazine 6mg PO or 5mg SC prn up to 8-hourly
Vestibular apparatus H$_1$, Ach$_m$	Tumours, motion	Hyoscine hydrobromide TD 1mg/72h or cyclizine 50mg 8-hourly	No dose reduction	Cyclizine 50mg prn 8-hourly	The alternative 1st-line drug

Specific drugs or effects required	Causes or indications	1st-line	Use in ESRD	prn drug	2nd-line
Prokinetic D2 Gastroparesis gastro-oesophageal reflux caused by	Drugs: opioids, NSAIDs, TCAs Diabetic neuropathy	Metoclopramide 10mg PO/SC tds before meals	50% normal dose; maximum 40mg/24h	Haloperidol 0.5mg up to 5mg/24h	Domperidone 20–20mg tds or 30mg PR bd
Antisecretory drugs	Bowel obstruction, colic	Hyoscine butylbromide	No dose reduction	Hyoscine butylbromide maximum 240mg/24h	Ocreotide doses 250–500mcg SC od in SD
5HT₃ receptor antagonists.* Present CTZ & vomiting centre	Chemo- or radiotherapy postoperative	Granisetron 1–2mg od, ondansetron 4–8mg bd, tropisetron 5mg od	Discontinue if ineffective after 3 days		May be enhanced by steroids. Late chemotherapy nausea or vomiting; consider levomepromazine as above

Abbreviations. Ach_m, muscarinic, cholinergic; CTZ, chemoreceptor trigger zone; D2, dopamine receptor; H₁, histamine type 1; od, once a day; PO, oral; prn, as required; TCA, tricyclic antidepressant; SL, sublingual; SC, subcutaneous; SD, syringe driver; TD, transdermal; tds, three times a day, 5HT₂, 5-hydroxytryptamine 2; 5HT₃, 5-hydroxytryptamine 3.

NB. Use and route for haloperidol outside terms of licence though widely used and recommended in palliative care practice.

* 5HT₃ receptor antagonists licensed for postoperative and chemo- and radiotherapy induce vomiting only.

Cautions. (1) Antimuscarinics block the final common (cholinergic) pathway through which prokinetic agents act: the two types of drugs, e.g. cyclizine and metoclopramide, should not be prescribed concurrently. (2) You should not use two antimuscarinic drugs together. (3) Antimuscarinics relax the lower oesophageal sphincter and, if possible, should be avoided in patients with symptomatic acid reflux.

Constipation

- Is also common.
- Multifactorial in origin. The following contribute in many patients.
  - Low roughage diet.
  - Reduced fluid intake.
  - Poor mobility.
  - Medication, e.g. oral iron, phosphate binders.
  - More common if on PD.

Management of constipation

General measures will be used according to appropriateness of the clinical situation.

- Increased fluid intake.
- High fibre diet.
- Increased mobility.
- Privacy and comfort during defecation.

Laxatives

Generally classified as stimulant or bulk forming, both are usually needed in the multifactorial origin of constipation in this population. Individual dose titration to benefit usually necessary.

- Stimulants.
  - Senna.
  - Bisacodyl.
  - Danthron (available as co danthramer and codanthrusate with softener—cause discoloration of the urine and should be avoided if incontinence because both urine and faeces can cause skin excoriation). Only licensed for the terminally ill in UK.

Stimulants must be accompanied with a softening laxative if stools hard; these include osmotic agents

- Softening agents.
  - Docusate, often used in conjunction with stimulant such as senna or combined preparation such as codanthrusate.
  - Macrogols such as polyethylene glycol. Contain the necessary water within the dispensed agent, so do not necessitate further water consumption, which may be difficult at end of life.
  - The sodium content of polyethylene glycol is safe for renal patients as it is not absorbed, but remains in the bowel.

Impaction can be treated with up to 8 sachets a day of polyethylene glycol. However, this is unlikely to be tolerable for someone at the end of life and rectal measures may be less exhausting and more comfortable.

Rectal measures

May be necessary to initiate return to regular bowel function.

- Glycerol suppository is stimulant and provides a faecal lubricant that aids evacuation through softening the stool.
- Bisacodyl suppositories are stimulant. They should touch the rectal mucosa and have effect within about an hour.

- Enemas will be needed for more intractable constipation or faecal impaction.
- Arachis oil enema is used to soften the stool. It is often given overnight followed by a phosphate enema in the morning.
  (NB. Arachis oil contains peanuts.)

Insomnia

Sleep disturbance and poor sleep probably affect up to half of dialysis patients though many will not mention it unless specifically asked. Sleep may be disturbed by other symptoms such as restless legs, pain, or cramps. In addition, patients may have sleep disorders such as sleep apnoea. Someone who is lethargic and inactive by day is likely to find it harder to sleep at night. Poor sleep and increased daytime sleepiness is known to be associated with reduced quality of life, emphasizing the importance of trying to help patients with this symptom. Characteristically the patient may complain of difficulty initiating sleep, early morning waking, or feeling unrefreshed in the morning. Insomnia is likely to be associated with many other symptoms, some of which may contribute to the cause and others that are a consequence of it, though the relationship can be difficult to unravel in symptoms such as daytime sleepiness.

Associations with insomnia

- Pain.
- Restless legs.
- Cramps.
- Depression.
- Lethargy due to anaemia, poor dialysis prescription, electrolyte disturbance.

Management considerations

- Consider and treat any reversible conditions:
  - pain;
  - other non-renal specific symptoms impacting on sleep;
  - itch;
  - restless legs;
  - anxiety, depression;
  - anaemia.
- Encourage good sleep hygiene.
- Psychological support possibly with relaxation techniques.
- Hypnotics.
  - Use at end of life should not be restricted, though earlier in the course of illness greater attention given to other means of alleviating the symptom.
  - Increased sensitivity to benzodiazepines in renal patients suggests one uses the shortest-acting hypnotics to try to prevent daytime sleepiness the following day.
  - Zopiclone and zolpidem recommended. Half-life 2–5h; act on same receptors as the benzodiazepines though pharmacologically different.

Restless legs syndrome (RLS)

RLS is defined as a sensory syndrome with a persistent and extremely uncomfortable 'crawling' sensation in the lower limbs. It is more prominent at night-time, may be sufficiently intense to interfere with sleep, and can often only be relieved by moving the extremities. The diagnosis is based on the patient's history.

Incidence Estimates in the general population suggest an incidence of 2–15% while studies of patients with ESRD show an incidence of 20–30% of patients with the lower incidence in the more rigorous studies. Primary RLS has a genetic origin; that seen in ESRD is secondary to a number of factors.

Pathophysiology The pathogenesis of RLS is not fully worked out but appears to involve dopaminergic dysfunction, iron metabolism, and abnormalities in supraspinal inhibition. It is postulated that RLS may be a form of uraemic neuropathy in ESRD patients.

Factors associated with its incidence
- Number of comorbidities.
- Anaemia.
- Low ferritin.
- Low parathyroid hormone levels.
- Inadequate dialysis.
- Longer period on dialysis.
- Pruritus.
- Age.
- Diabetes mellitus.
- Medication, e.g. tricyclic antidepressants, caffeine, neuroleptics.

Effect of RLS It is associated with poor sleep and daytime lethargy, an impaired quality of life, and an increased risk of death. There is a suggestion in one study that it is associated with premature cessation of dialysis, though this may be due to its other associations rather than a direct relationship with RLS. Vigorous management is important to try to restore sleep and an improvement in quality of life.

General management considerations
- Adequate dialysis if appropriate.
- Avoidance of precipitating medication.
- Treatment of anaemia, as appropriate to stage of illness.

Pharmacological treatment
There are very few studies comparing different drug regimens with each other in patients with ESRD. Careful dose titration needs to take place for each patient. The rank in which drugs are tried will depend on stage of disease.

- Dopamine receptor agonist therapy, including pramipexole, ropinirole, pergolide, or cabergoline, may be considered as the first-line treatment for RLS. All need slow titration, however.
  - Adverse effects such as daytime sleepiness and augmentation may limit their use particularly at the end of life.
- Benzodiazepines may give more immediate relief, are easy to titrate, and are more appropriate at end of life.
  - Useful if RLS causing sleep disturbance.
  - Clonazepam suggested starting dose: 500–1000mcg at night.
  - Must monitor benzodiazepines because of increased sensitivity.
- Anticonvulsants such as gabapentin have been used—must remember appropriate dose adjustments. See Table 15.2, p. 283.
- Opioids; some emerging evidence in non-renal patients; the usual opioid restrictions would apply but may consider their use in refractory cases.

Symptoms from long-term complications of treatment of ESRD

The long-term complications of treated end-stage renal disease lead to renal-specific complications such as the deposition of amyloid particularly in joints or renal osteodystrophy. Sexual disorders occur in many other conditions but there are factors in renal failure that lead to the high incidence in many renal patients. Cramps, too, are common in the general population but of increased incidence particularly during dialysis. Joint and other pain management is considered in Chapter 6.

Calciphylaxis

Calciphylaxis is a syndrome where there is calcification of small arteries and subcutaneous tissues, as a consequence of secondary hyperparathyroidism. This can lead to severe pain from ischaemic skin ulceration. It is associated with a very poor prognosis and has a high mortality. The patient often has a reduced performance status with a gradual physical deterioration. Other effects of ischaemia may also be present with complications of peripheral vascular disease.

Management considerations

- The main symptom from this extremely unpleasant complication of ESRD is pain both in the ulcerated area and increased sensitivity of affected but as yet unbroken skin. Pain management is considered in detail in Chapter 6. Pain is usually both nociceptive and neuropathic in nature, requiring intense management particularly as the patient's clinical condition may change frequently with overall deterioration.
- Management of the skin ulceration—see p. 140.
- Psychosocial support to someone with increasing dependence and physical disfigurement requiring painful dressing changes and whose prognosis is severely limited.
- It is important to enable patients to have a discussion about the prognostic implications of this diagnosis in a supportive environment.

Cramps

Muscle cramps, defined as an involuntary and forcibly contracted muscle, are extremely common particularly in the elderly. They occur more frequently in dialysis patients both in relation to the dialysis procedure or immediately after it with a frequency in one study of greater than 50%.

Cramps are associated with imbalances of water and electrolytes (particularly sodium calcium, magnesium, and potassium). The exact aetiology in relation to dialysis is not fully understood but it seems reasonable to assume that it is a secondary effect of the removal of water and solutes. There seems to be a direct relationship between the volume of fluid removed and development of dialysis-related cramps. In addition, in the person with normal renal function they are known to be associated with muscle fatigue.

Management strategies
Physical help with muscle stretching or application of warmth may be sufficient. Drug therapy if needed will depend on stage of disease.
- If on dialysis:
  - adjustment of dialysis sodium and potassium;
  - carnitine during dialysis.
- End of life:
  - quinine;
  - vitamin E 400IU orally.

Sexual disorders and problems

Both men and women with chronic kidney disease experience sexual dysfunction with both experiencing decreased libido and reduced sexual arousal and reduced fertility. Men commonly report erectile dysfunction and women pain during intercourse and difficulty achieving orgasm. The severity of symptoms does not relate to duration of CKD or type of dialysis, and some symptoms pre-date the diagnosis.

The causes relate both to hormone changes, such as reduced testosterone or ovarian failure in women, and to patients' underlying diseases such as diabetes and peripheral vascular disease.

At end of life these symptoms may reduce in significance but may have affected physical intimacy earlier on in the illness. This may impact on the relationship between patient and their partner at end of life. It is essential to remember the importance of privacy for patients at end of life to enable there to be intimacy if wished as many will not ask.

Symptoms related to comorbid conditions

Neuropathy (non-pain manifestations)

The commonest cause of neuropathy in CKD patients is diabetic neuropathy, manifesting itself most usually as either gastroparesis or enteropathy or both.

Diabetic gastroparesis

Delayed gastric emptying is common in CKD, with several other contributing factors including drugs and renal failure itself. Gastric emptying studies are needed to confirm the diagnosis of diabetic gastroparesis, which leads to anorexia, early satiety, nausea, vomiting, and weight loss.

Management
- Optimal management of diabetes.
- Frequent small meals, minimizing hyperglycaemia (may not be appropriate at end of life).
- Prokinetic agents; see Table 7.2, p. 131.
- Erythromycin only in cases of intractable symptoms where potential for ill effects counterbalanced by possible efficacy.
- Acid suppression may also be considered either with proton pump inhibitor or H_2 blocker.

Diabetic enteropathy

A disorder characterized by diarrhoea alternating with constipation. The former may be painless, watery, occur without warning, and cause incontinence. Probable pathogenic mechanisms include abnormal motility and bacterial overgrowth.

Management

At end of life treatment is geared to relief of symptoms. Codeine is best avoided in view of possible toxicity.
- Symptomatic treatment of diarrhoea with loperamide.
- Supportive management of incontinence.

Other autonomic symptoms may occur such as loss of temperature regulation, sweating, and hypotension. Some of these symptoms will become less prominent at end of life but others need to be kept in mind when caring for the dying patient as symptomatic treatment may need to continue to maintain comfort.

Peripheral vascular disease (PVD) This is described in detail in Chapter 2. The main symptoms are pain from skin ischaemia, claudication, or ischaemic ulceration and phantom limb pain if amputation is necessary. When these complications start to occur this is often an indication that prognosis is short. See Chapter 6 for pain management and below for treatment of ulceration.

Ischaemic heart disease This is described in Chapter 2 (p. 20). Symptoms such as angina, flash pulmonary oedema, and hypotension may continue in the terminal phase and need ongoing management.

Other skin problems

Diabetic foot

The common combination of PVD and diabetes with peripheral neuropathy and reduced sensation in the foot can lead to severe symptoms from gangrene or non-healing ulcers, both of which can be very painful. Ongoing consideration of this to ensure maximum comfort at end of life will be important.

Decubitus ulcers

Factors that predispose to pressure ulcers include:
- immobility;
- poor nutritional status with low albumin;
- infection;
- incontinence;
- oedema.

These factors are present in many ESRD patients as they approach the end of their lives and their effect is added to by uraemia and the necessity of transportation and manual handling for dialysis. Prevention is the most important aspect of their management, which requires excellent nursing care. The occurrence of ulcers despite proper skin care reflects the advanced state of ill health and may be indicative of closeness to death.

Management

Is geared towards comfort. It is unlikely that healing will be achieved, but important to prevent extension of ulceration where possible and ensure comfort. Details of care will depend on the presence or absence of:
- exudate;
- bleeding;
- necrotic tissue;
- odour;
- infection;
- cosmesis.

Pain management during dressing change is extremely important and considered under procedure-related pain management and topical opioids in Chapter 6 (pp. 106–8).

Skin and ulcer care will depend on stage of illness and includes:
- establishing the goal of treatment, i.e. comfort or cure;
- attention to pressure-relieving mattress;
- good skin hygiene;
- prevention of pressure from overlying bed clothes;
- assessment and record of type of wound.

Dialysis-related symptoms

Cramps Discussed on p. 138, these can sometimes be extremely severe during dialysis. For some patients they occur during most dialysis sessions.

Hypotension

Hypotension may occur both early and late during dialysis and lead to unpleasant symptoms for the patient during dialysis that make the procedure difficult to tolerate. It is always important to assess the fluid status of the patient and give fluids if the patient is thought to be hypovolaemic. Hypotension on dialysis is more common in patients with large weight gains requiring greater fluid removal during dialysis, and in patients with poor cardiac function. The use of haemodiafiltration in patients with poor cardiac function may result in less hypotension. There is a significant risk of cardiac arrest in patients who are hypotensive at the start of dialysis and this may be a reason for considering withdrawal of dialysis (if there are no reversible features).

Other symptoms

Depression

Depression is common in ESRD patients. Its prevalence is difficult to quantify as many of its symptoms are similar to those of chronic renal disease. However, it is thought that up to one in five ESRD patients suffer a major depression and about twice that number depressive symptoms. It is associated with pain, insomnia, fatigue, and anorexia and it is not always possible to determine which symptom came first as all the associated symptoms have a high incidence in renal patients. Diagnosis may be difficult because the somatic symptoms may have other causes. Where there is difficulty in making a diagnosis, use of the Cognitive Depression Inventory within the Beck Depression Inventory may be helpful as this concentrates on guilt, sadness, and difficulty in making decisions rather than somatic symptoms. Key stages of disease progression or increase in complications, including the recognition that the end of life may be close in someone's renal history, are likely to be times of increased risk of depression. For someone who has been struggling with dialysis and who has recognized and accepted their own mortality, the cessation of dialysis may bring relief of depression.

Management issues at end of life

- Psychosocial and spiritual support to patient and family in combination with drugs targeting the main manifestation of the depression will be needed at end of life.
- If anxiety chief manifestation then anxiolytic therapy (see below) may give rapid relief.
- Similarly it may be used for agitated depression.
- Insomnia should be addressed vigorously as improvement may lift mood.
  - Tricyclic antidepressants may be used for hypnotic effect if also indicated for neuropathic pain.

Antidepressants

May not have time to be effective. Most are fat-soluble, easily pass the blood–brain barrier, are not dialysable, are metabolized primarily by the liver, and are excreted mainly in bile. Consequently, the majority of these drugs can be safely used in this population.

- Tricyclic antidepressants are as effective as in the general population but may be contraindicated because of side-effect profile. However, may be considered for their hypnotic effect or for severe depression. They should be started at low dose and titrated upward according to response and if no toxicity.
  - Amitryptyline: dose modification not necessary but side-effects likely to limit use and dose achievable.
- Serotonin re-uptake inhibitors (SSRIs) that can be used without dose modification include citalopram, fluoxetene, and sertraline.

Anxiety

Anxiety is also common. It is to be expected that its presence and severity will fluctuate during the course of the renal illness, as patients adjust to a different set of norms for their own functioning and dependence. Again symptoms may mimic those from uraemia. It is important for staff to recognize anxiety and stress, to allow time for their expression which may be therapeutic, and to refer on those whose symptoms are very severe or disabling.

Pharmacological management

May be necessary where symptoms are severe or disabling. The mainstay of treatment is benzodiazepines, though SSRIs may be used for panic or general anxiety disorders.

- Diazepam. Ordinary doses can be used, but it accumulates in normal renal function and active metabolites in ESRD, so monitoring and dose reduction will become necessary.
- Midazolam given SC is useful for rapid onset and short duration at end of life. It can also be given in a syringe driver for more prolonged use (see Chapter 12). Dose reduction is necessary because of prolongation of half-life in the over-60s and because active metabolites accumulate in renal impairment.
- Lorazepam can be given PO, SL, or IV but not SC. It has a rapid onset of action, and is useful for panic attacks. However, it too accumulates in renal failure so care should be taken with repeated doses.

Symptoms associated with end of life The occurrence and management of symptoms such as dyspnoea, confusion, and agitation that are more commonly associated with the terminal phase are described in Chapter 12.

Summary

Extremely ill dialysis patients, those who opt not to dialyse, and those who stop dialysis have a significant symptom burden that impacts on their quality of life. Many of these patients may benefit from more aggressive treatment of their symptoms, which could include support from a palliative care team while continuing under the care of their nephrologist to ensure optimal management of the renal condition. Recognition of the problem through the use of simple assessment measures with guidelines to promote good practice may improve the overall care of these patients and particularly those approaching the end of their lives.

Further reading

Weisbord SD, Carmody SS, Gruns FJ, *et al.* (2003). Symptom burden, quality of life, advance care planning and the potential value of palliative care in severely ill haemodialysis patients. *Nephrol Dial Transplant* **18**, 1345–52.

Murtagh FE, Addington-Hall JM, Donohoe P, *et al.* (2006). Symptom management in patients with established renal failure managed without dialysis. *EDTNA ERCA J* **32** (2), 93–8,

Recognizing dying

Introduction

In order to provide the best possible care for someone at the end of their life it is important to identify that they have reached an irreversible stage in their illness. This is particularly difficult in people with a chronic illness who experience a slow decline. It might be helpful to address it in two stages:

• recognition of the need for supportive and palliative care;
• recognition of the terminal phase—meaning the last days and weeks of life.

Recognition of the need for supportive and palliative care

There are a number of markers that will help the clinician realize that their patient is in need of supportive care, particularly if one uses a modification of the 1990 WHO definition of palliative care substituting renal patient for cancer patient.

The active total care of patients whose disease is not responsive to curative treatment. Control of pain, of other symptoms, and of psychological, social, and spiritual problems is paramount. The goal of palliative care is achievement of the best quality of life for patients and their families. Many aspects of palliative care are also applicable earlier in the course of the illness **in conjunction with conventional care for the renal patient**

Modified from WHO 1990

One helpful way to raise awareness in one's own practice is to ask the question 'Would you be surprised if this person were to die in the next 12 months?' If the answer is 'no', the clinician should be considering if such a person has palliative care needs. Prognostication is a very inexact science. However, we know that clinicians overestimate prognosis more frequently than the converse. Therefore, if in doubt, the chances are the person does have a prognosis of less that 12 months. In the UK a general practice initiative called the Gold Standards Framework can help both identify patients and then improve their care.

Gold Standards Framework (GSF)

The aim of the GSF is to provide one **gold standard** for all end of life care. It is a programme for community palliative care, practice- or locality-based. It has a common sense framework that was initially developed for cancer care but is now recognized to be relevant to all with supportive and palliative care needs aiming to optimize the organization of and the quality of care. The key elements all involve communication and are patient-centred.

- Identify patients in need of palliative/supportive care.
- Assess their needs, symptoms, preferences.
- Plan care around needs.

The goals of care are that the patient:
- is **symptom-free** or at minimum has symptoms addressed;
- identifies their **preferred place of end of life care**;
- feels **secure and supported** by means of:
  - advance care planning;
  - addressing information needs;
  - knowledge that planned care will lead to fewer crisis admissions.

For carers and staff the gains are as follows.
- Carers are supported, enabled, and empowered to provide optimal care.
- Staff gain confidence through team working.

The seven Cs
The GSF identifies key tasks, known as the 'seven Cs'.
- **Communication** within primary care which includes:
  - a register of all patients with palliative care needs;
  - all such patients discussed at a multidisciplinary meeting;
  - improved discussion with patient to include advance care planning.
- **Coordination** of care with nomination of a co-coordinator.
- **Control of symptoms,** which should be:
  - assessed;
  - recorded;
  - acted on.
- **Continuity,** which includes out of hours care (OOH):
  - systems put in place for OOH care.
- **Continued learning** by primary care.
- **Carer support**.
- **Care of the dying** phase:
  - diagnosing dying;
  - could use integrated care pathway (see Chapter 12, p. 252);
  - must use anticipatory prescribing.

Prognostic indicator
To aid the identification of adult patients with advanced disease, in the last months or year of life, and those who are in need of supportive and palliative care a **prognostic indicator** is being developed. This encompasses the following.

General predictors of end-stage disease

- Multiple comorbidities (with no primary diagnosis).
- Weight loss: greater than 10% weight loss over 6 months.
- General physical decline.
- Serum albumin < 25g/L.
- Reduced performance status/Karnofsky performance score (KPS) < 50%.
- Dependence in most activities of daily living (ADL).

Indicators specific to renal disease

- Conservative care: patients with stage 5 CKD who are not seeking dialysis or are discontinuing it and are not for renal transplant. Reasons include:
  - personal choice;
  - frailty or the presence of too many comorbid conditions.
- Patients with stage 4 or 5 CKD whose condition is deteriorating and for whom the '1-year surprise question' is applicable, i.e. overall you would not be surprised if they were to die in the next year.
- Clinical indicators:
  - CKD stage 5 (estimated GFR < 15mL/min);
  - symptomatic renal failure (anorexia, nausea, pruritus, reduced functional status, intractable fluid overload).

Indicators taken from GSF prognostic indicator guidance.[1]

Reference

1 The gold standards framework NHS End of Life Programme: *www.goldstandardsframework.nhs.uk*

Recognition of the terminal phase

Clinical practice

In the context of patients seen in outpatients or on the renal wards there are a number of factors that lead clinicians to recognize the approach of end of life.

- A rapid change in performance status with:
  - increasing dependence;
  - more time spent in bed.
- Weight loss with cachexia in the absence of malignancy.
- Multiple admissions with complications of treatment.
- Increasing difficulty with access for dialysis.
- Irreversibility of comorbid conditions such as:
  - worsening peripheral vascular disease not amenable to corrective surgery and leading to amputations;
  - ongoing complications of vasculopathy, either cardiac, cerebral, or gut ischaemia.
- Calciphylaxis—usually associated with a poor prognosis.
- Recurrent infections.
- Increasingly severe symptoms, needing more complex management.
- Patient withdrawal from interest in the world around them. This may take various forms:
  - refusal of food and drink;
  - refusal of medication;
  - refusal of basic nursing care;
  - irritability with staff who are trying to help them.

If the patient declines dialysis then it is possible to open a discussion with them to check their understanding of the consequences of their decision and then support them through the consequences of their choice.

Refusal of other care but not dialysis is often a cry for help, perhaps by someone who cannot verbalize their feelings, and it should be seen as an opportunity for gentle exploration to determine the patient's wishes and fears, and also to exclude depression or another cause that might be responsive to treatment.

Clinicians will always wish to ensure that no reversible causes of some of the above factors are missed. However, it is often helpful to discuss with the patient to what lengths they wish to go with investigations if the cause of decline is unclear. Without taking away hope it is possible to share with the patient your concern that not all illnesses are reversible and then to ask their view on how far they wish to be investigated balancing the burden against benefit. There will be some who have recognized already that their prognosis is now limited and others who come to recognize that the situation is irreversible. Both are then likely to welcome the opportunity to discuss options in an honest and open fashion—perhaps to stop fighting and concentrate efforts on quality of life within the constraints of their illness. Others will wish you to use all reasonable resources to try to improve the situation.

If a patient is experiencing pain or other distressing symptoms, whatever the uncertainty about their prognosis, it is important to provide meticulous symptom control. If that person dies, you have provided the right kind of care for their end of life. If they survive, you will have improved their quality of life during a difficult time.

Listening to the patient and their families/carers

As well as the patient recognizing that they are approaching the end of their lives, often the family or carers suspect or are concerned that their relative is moving towards the final stage of their illness. It is vital that patients, families, and carers feel able to express their concerns to any member of the renal team, who should ensure that there are opportunities to look at the whole situation for an individual not just the care necessary for their renal disease. These opportunities can be provided in a variety of ways such as access to non-medical members of the team who can feed back to a multidisciplinary meeting. A regular overall assessment at dialysis attendance could include an open question asking how things are, which would give patients the opportunity to say if they are struggling.

The patient and family perspective

'I thought I would walk out of here on two feet but now I am not so sure'

Patients come to the realization that they are dying in their own time and in their own way with a range of emotions and coping strategies accompanying this recognition. Worden's work on loss in the context of mourning explains the emotions patients experience as they are confronted with their own mortality and their passage through overlapping stages of coping from the time that they become aware of their prognosis until their actual death.[1] In order to be of help, we must first appreciate the enormous psychological impact dying has on the terminally ill patient and his family. Insight into the nature and range of coping mechanisms patients employ to manage the many powerful and sometimes conflicting emotions elicited by the prospect of death is paramount, as only by understanding this model of grief are we able to share the patient's unique journey and offer the most appropriate intervention. Patients express loss in different ways, rarely if ever progressing systematically through the stages of mourning but more frequently dipping in and out as they process newly acquired information. At such times it is helpful if their behaviour and emotions can be normalized within the framework of someone who is grieving not just for what they have lost, but also anticipatory grief for what they are about to lose.

Most commonly expressed emotions at this time are:
- denial;
- anger and despair that, if internalized, can manifest as depression;
- difficulty in making decisions about future care pathways;
- sadness that life is to end and goodbyes need to be said;
- fear about the process of dying;
- anxiety about those left behind and any business left unfinished;
- ambivalence;

- guilt and self reproach—wondering if a change of lifestyle could have prevented progression of the disease;
- isolation, often self-imposed, as a sense of 'aloneness' encompasses them;
- helplessness and powerlessness—at not being able to change the inevitable course that their illness will take;
- yearning for what was and what will never again be;
- relief that the struggle will soon be over;
- acceptance that death is inevitable.

Reference

1 Worden JW (1991). *Grief counseling and grief therapy*. Springer, New York.

The nephrologist's perspective

It is as important to diagnose and appropriately manage the terminal phase of the patient's illness as it is to diagnose and treat a chest infection. Nephrologists, however, often find this difficult. There are various reasons for this.

- Patients can often be temporarily 'rescued' by yet another vascular access procedure.
- Patients are often referred from other teams when they develop acute renal failure as a complication of other severe illness or after surgery.
  - There is often an expectation from referring team, patient, and/or relatives that 'something can be done'.
  - Tendency to focus on 'here and now' and not long-term situation.
  - Difficult to be person to say 'no' to further intervention when referring team should have recognized futility of escalating treatment.
- Many nephrologists are not adequately trained to share bad news with patients and are therefore hesitant about having such conversations.
- In many renal units, patients are admitted on to the wards under the care of a nephrologist different to the one responsible for their usual care on the dialysis unit or in the transplant clinic. Understandably it is difficult to have 'end of life' discussions between a patient and an unknown doctor.
- Having such conversations is time-consuming.
- Many patients with ESRD are from ethnic minorities and speak poor English; this makes communication difficult.
- Nephrologists often work in rotation, i.e. may be 'on the wards' for a fixed period of time and then hand over to a colleague. In such a system, it is easy not to confront the difficult decisions.

Difficult questions about dialysis at end of life

- Is resuscitation always appropriate?
- Is transfer from PD to HD in weeks leading to death appropriate?
- Is perseverance with HD in patient tolerating dialysis poorly justified?
- Are multiple attempts at catheter insertion appropriate at end of life?

Clinicians should bear these questions in mind as they care for the very sick patient who may be near the end of their life and use this as an opportunity to raise their concerns sensitively with them. See Chapter 9.

Withdrawal of dialysis

- Difficult area to explore with patient but not uncommon for patients to recognize futility of treatment
- Indicated if high risk of patient having a cardiac arrest during a dialysis or dying while on the machine
- Effectively necessary if no further dialysis access possible

Communicating with patients and families

Deciding not to start dialysis

Good communication is the bridge that spans the gap between the mind of the doctor and the patient

Anna Tharyan

Margaret was a 61-year-old married patient with type II diabetes, partial vision, neuropathy, and CKD. Her quality of life had been substantially affected by her deteriorating renal function and she was dependent upon her husband for assistance with personal care and activities of daily living. Her own child had died 3 years previously from CKD having asked to be withdrawn from dialysis and Margaret's decision not to initiate treatment was based on her daughter's negative experience of renal replacement therapy, her unwillingness to integrate another health regime into her daily routine, and fear of becoming a further burden on her husband who had his own health problems. This, combined with issues around unresolved grief in relation to the death of her daughter, made her feel that the future held nothing for her.

Information gathering

Some patients make decisions not to embark upon dialysis as they feel it will offer no appreciable improvement to their quality of life and that it will impose unacceptable restrictions on them. In such instances it is essential that we are reassured that they fully understand the implications of their decision. Asking your patient 'what do you understand about how your disease will progress should you elect not to have dialysis?' enables the professional to know what the patient's understanding is and is also a stepping stone to discussions around end of life care.

Taking the conversation forward

Having ascertained that the patient realizes the consequences of not starting dialysis you can take the conversation forward to include discussion about sources of support and preferences for end of life care.

- 'Electing not to have dialysis doesn't mean you won't receive ongoing management of your kidney disease to keep you as well as we can, including treatment for any symptoms. It might be that you would like to have some local support in addition to the renal clinic such as the local community palliative care service.'
- 'You have said that you understand your lifespan might well be reduced as a result of your decision not to start dialysis and I wonder if now is the right time to look at where you would like to be cared for when your condition worsens.'

If the patient is happy to carry on with the conversation you could continue as follows.

● 'The options you might want to consider and discuss with your family include remaining at home, being cared for in hospital, or hospice admission. Talking about these now will help us plan things to try to ensure your wishes are carried out.'

Saying this reassures the patient that they are not going to be abandoned as a result of choosing the 'no dialysis treatments' option and empowers them to participate in decisions regarding end of life care and their preferred place of death.

Knowing what to ask and when is very dependent upon the relationship that has been built up with the patient or family member but, by active listening, cues can be picked up from the patient as to whether they are ready to 'hear' what is being said.

● 'You mentioned that you don't want dialysis treatment and realize that you might die sooner rather than later without it. We want to be able to offer you consistent care throughout the period of your conservative management and I wonder if you want to look at the support that can be on offer to you now and later?'

It should be remembered that when a patient makes a decision not to have dialysis, they could still live for several months. Looking at end of life care and preferred place of death may not be uppermost in the patient's mind for they still consider that they have a life to live.

However, for patients facing death more imminently, these issues have to be gently raised.

● 'You say you are becoming more symptomatic and that you have no quality of life to speak of. Can you tell me what you are finding difficult to manage at home and whether you need to be considering accepting help in order to remain there or has the time now come for you to look at other options?'

This approach hands back the decision-making to the patient leaving them feeling in control even though their life is out of control.

Broaching palliative and hospice care

It should be borne in mind that many patients regard hospices as 'somewhere you go to die' and there is often resistance to onward referral for hospice end of life care. This can be helped by introducing such care through the more generic term 'palliative care' and then explaining that hospice care is part of palliative care, having explained a little of the philosophy of palliative care.

Depending on where the patient is in their understanding, it can be useful to say the following.

• 'I want to reassure you that I am not raising the subject of palliative care because I have concerns about your immediate health, I just want you to be aware that we often make early referrals to hospice and palliative care services because they offer a different dimension to the care we can give you. Nurses can visit and advise on symptom management and are available as a resource, particularly if you want to take advantage of the day care facilities and therapies they offer. They also provide emotional support, not only to patients but also to family members, and maybe this is something you would find useful at some time in the future.'

Educating patients as to the resources that are available within hospice and palliative care services can address verbalized resistance and lead to the terminally ill patient and family members benefiting from local support services. See also Chapter 10.

Helping with decision-making

An increasing number of patients postpone making decisions regarding future treatment plans based on their assertion that they aren't symptomatic and therefore there is no urgency. Whilst not wanting to pressure ambivalent patients, it can be helpful to say the following.

- 'I can see that it is difficult to make a decision about future treatment options when you are not experiencing any symptoms, but sometimes, despite being closely monitored, things change suddenly and then immediate decisions have to be taken as to whether or not to start dialysis. This could lead to you being treated in a way you would not have chosen. So if you are able to make a firm decision you are ensuring that the care you receive will be in line with your wishes.'

However, it is also important to reassure patients that we recognize that they may change their minds when the clinical situation changes. This can be acknowledged by reassuring them as follows.

- 'We recognize that sometimes when circumstances change people do rethink their decisions and there will be the chance for further discussion in the future.'

Avoidance techniques

We also need to remain aware that avoidant behaviour and denial are commonly expressed defence mechanisms that some patients employ at this stage of their illness, which is why decision-making can be such a difficult task. It is not unusual for patients to say 'I'll do whatever the doctor thinks I should do' rather than take responsibility for their future care. We need to appreciate the internal conflict patients often experience at this time and sensitively find ways of addressing their dilemmas.

Following reflection

And, finally, we should remember that in this situation patients do quite often change their minds. As they become more symptomatic, so are they more likely to see dialysis as a means of reducing their symptoms and improving their health and quality of life. This is why it is important for a member of the renal team to continue to see these patients to offer them the opportunity to re-think their original decision, and to give them permission to change their mind.

Withdrawal from dialysis

> Adjustment to death is a process that cannot be rushed

Informed decision-making regarding stopping dialysis

Dialysis, especially haemodialysis, can be a stressful and exhausting regime particularly for elderly patients or those with comorbidities. When dialysis is no longer seen as maintaining or improving quality of life, or indeed is causing the patient distress, patients and family members might be offered a discussion about withdrawing from dialysis. Conversely, some patients may make a conscious decision to withdraw from treatment, in which case discussions with the medical team and family members should take place to explore the reasons behind this request or whether any changes in treatment might improve quality of life before a final decision is made about stopping treatment. It is imperative that any questions raised by the patient and family members are honestly addressed in order that informed decisions can be made and future care plans put in place. See also Chapters 11 and 12.

It is essential for patients to understand the following.

- Informed decision-making will be respected.
- Open and honest dialogue will take place with the medical staff acting as 'facilitators' if the patient is experiencing difficulty discussing this option with family members.
- A psychological assessment may be required:
  - if the decision to withdraw is made for solely emotional reasons; *or*
  - there is evidence of depression that could be treated with medication or counselling, which might change the patient's perspective;
  - to establish that the patient has made an informed decision to withdraw and fully understands the implications and consequences of that decision.
- Time for reflection is encouraged.
- Treatment can be reinstated if the patient so wishes.

It is equally important that staff remember that the wishes of a patient who is able to make an informed decision should take precedence over all other considerations and that withdrawal from dialysis can offer patients a chance of taking control over the final days of their lives.

From the example of Mimi in the box opposite, it can be seen that many personal, family, and social factors contribute towards the decision to withdraw from treatment. These need to be understood by staff in order to appreciate the patient's dilemmas and difficulties. Support needs to be offered to both patients and their families at such times.

Mimi was 82 years old, widowed, with one married son. She lived alone and was mentally alert but physically struggling to manage daily living and personal care tasks. No longer able to carry out PD she found the rigours of HD difficult to tolerate and asked that treatment be withdrawn. Her son offered to pay for her to move into a nursing home where she could recommence PD, but she refused saying she wanted to live with him—something his wife refused to consider. Conservative management was gently introduced as a treatment option and Mimi agreed that this would be her preferred course of action. However, within the next 2 weeks, she repeatedly vacillated, which resulted in treatment being recommenced and withdrawn three times. Her son thought her indecisiveness was aimed at making him feel guilty but in discussion with her it became clear that she had huge fears around death and dying—particularly the time frame and way in which death from renal failure would occur. Mimi was referred to both the hospital chaplain and the counsellor and died peacefully in hospital, but her son, who had stopped visiting because he found it too painful, sought emotional support for several months following her death

Helping families consider withdrawal from dialysis and palliative care

'I can't possibly make that decision—it's like I'm signing my father's death warrant'

One aspect of palliative care is that it can be seen as creating a voice for the voiceless, particularly when a person loses capacity. It is about recognizing that, when someone is ill and dying, they may be unable to voice what they want and how their needs can be met, which can leave families feeling that they are shouldering the responsibility of decision-making regarding withholding or withdrawal of dialysis.

A useful intervention and one which families would find more acceptable might be for medical staff to say 'In our opinion, dialysis is simply sustaining life; unfortunately your father is not going to improve and it is unlikely he will recover from the stroke. It is our clinical judgement that dialysis should be withdrawn and we were wondering if you feel able to support this decision?' Or 'If your father was able to speak what do you think he would be saying now? What do you imagine his wishes would be?'

Framed in this way, the onus of responsibility shifts and families feel better able to make decisions based on what they believe their loved ones would have wanted. See also Chapter 11.

Palliative care necessitates comprehensive caring and places a high priority on both physical and emotional comfort. Its objectives include the management of pain and other symptoms, diagnosis and treatment of psychological distress, and assistance in maintaining independence for as long as possible. It also extends to supporting the family. For further information see Chapter 10.

Raising awareness and improving communication skills

Improving communication can improve end of life care

Overview

Patients have identified fear of pain, loss of dignity, abandonment, and fear of the unknown as major concerns in relation to their own mortality and have cited six themes that they consider to be of importance when issues around death and dying are being discussed. These include:

- an honest and straightforward approach;
- sensitive handling of bad news;
- active listening to patients;
- encouragement of patients and relatives to ask questions;
- a willingness to talk about death and dying;
- attunement to patients by being prepared to be guided by them.

Conversely, studies of why doctors have difficulties in discussions with patients around the end of life highlight common issues:[1]

- personal discomfort with confronting mortality;
- fear of damaging the doctor–patient relationship or harming the patient by raising the topic of death;
- limited time to establish trust;
- difficulty in managing complex family dynamics;
- fear of being blamed.

An example of how not to communicate

Dr. X waited until my mother had left and then breezed in. He said 'Well things aren't going too well are they and I wonder if you have thought about going home to die, or perhaps going to a hospice?' I didn't think I had heard him right. I mean I know I have had an uphill struggle but I didn't think I was dying. I said 'Are you giving up on me then?' and he said that nutritionally I was in a bad way and that this affected the quality of the dialysis I was receiving which he knew I was finding difficult to tolerate—and he couldn't see me improving. I just lay there trying to gather my thoughts—wondering what I should say—when he turned tail and left saying 'give it some thought'. I was so shocked and upset that when my husband came in about half an hour later, I just sobbed and sobbed. I didn't want him to go home and the nurses put the camp bed up in my room for him to use. But I couldn't sleep because I was frightened I wouldn't wake up and I was sick three times—probably through anxiety. Why couldn't he have waited till my family was here and broken it to me more gently? I don't want to see him again'

Appreciation of where patients think they are in their illness can be established by exploring not only what they understand of their prognosis but how they are coping with it emotionally. What we say to patients and how the message is communicated can profoundly affect the way in which a patient deals with what they have heard. If done badly, it can also cause a breakdown in the doctor–patient relationship as the example in the box shows.

This hurried and insensitive discourse and the way in which the doctor quickly left the ward emphasized the inequality in the relationship in that he could literally move on whereas she couldn't—neither physically nor emotionally. No doubt he felt he had carried out his duty in discussing prognosis and future care, but where was his duty of care to this patient? She was left feeling abandoned, frightened, angry, confused, and vulnerable. Ideally, the doctor should have stayed with the sense of denial she held around her own mortality and helped her acclimatize and integrate the new reality, but perhaps his own discomfort around death and dying, his lack of expertise of sharing bad news with patient, together with feelings of failure at not being able to cure her, may have prevented this.

It is also worth remembering that we can close all channels of communication with the gesture of a hand or an inappropriate response. But they can be opened up through eye contact, hand gestures, touch, or by adopting a genuinely caring and concerned approach.

Good communication needs to cover strategies to alleviate patient and family distress and best practice dictates a more acceptable way of approaching this patient would have been to ensure that:

• the consultation was not rushed;
• a family member or the patient's named nurse was present;
• the clinician established the patient's understanding of the situation;
• an empathic, sensitive, and patient-centred approach was used;
• the patient was not told that nothing further could be done but reassured that, even if dialysis was withdrawn, symptoms would be managed;
• questions were encouraged and honestly answered;
• the expression of patient and family emotions were appropriately facilitated and referral for ongoing support offered if deemed necessary;
• withdrawal from treatment was explored and support networks provided if appropriate;
• prognostic time frames were given as accurately and honestly as possible, where requested, to enable realistic decision-making;
• further consultations were offered to define primary goals and address any unanswered questions.

Reference

1 Calam B, Far S, Andrew R (2000). Discussions of 'code status' on a family practice teaching ward: what barriers do family physicians face? *Can Med Assoc J* **163** (10), 1255–9.

Sharing bad news

An acceptable way of starting communication that imparts bad news is to first find out what the patient understands of their illness. This can be done with straightforward questioning, such as:

- 'Can you tell me what you understand of your illness and what might happen next?'

Having established the level of understanding, the new and undoubtedly distressing information needs to be shared.

- 'I am sorry to have to tell you…'
- 'Unfortunately it does look as though…'
- 'Tests would seem to indicate you have…'

For some patients, bad news comes as a relief—that at last their fears have been put into words. But it is also imperative to let the patient know that, whilst death is inevitable, treatment of some kind will continue.

- 'Whilst there is no curative treatment we can offer, your symptoms will be managed and your wishes regarding future care honoured.'

Effective communication comes through being comfortable with our own discomfort. For many people the thought of dying evokes even more anxiety and fear than the thought of death itself. Dying should not be a taboo subject and patients should be encouraged to talk about their limited future and consider how they want to live whilst waiting to die.

Effective communication can help allay fears, minimize pain and suffering, and enable patients and their families to experience a peaceful end to life. Avoid advising patients with 'shoulds', 'oughts', and 'musts' but invite them to reach their own understanding and decision-making by open and honest dialogue. This can be facilitated by questions such as 'Do you want me to tell you what is likely to happen now?' or 'Would you find it helpful if I told you how things might progress?'

Having established the patient's level of understanding, thought can then be given to the information that needs to be gathered in order to address any underlying concerns the patient may have and not be able to voice.

Gentle probing can usually elicit what the patient is thinking and feeling.

- 'Knowing what the situation is, what would you say are your major concerns and are there any further explanations I can give to help you resolve them?'
- 'Have you thought about how you will cope during this phase of your illness, and what support you might need?'
- 'How aware of the situation do you think your family is. Would you like me to speak to them or be available when you talk with them?'
- 'We can't always talk to our closest family for fear of upsetting them and I am wondering whom you can talk to about how you are feeling.'
- 'Is there anyone here you would find it easy to talk to?'
- 'Some patients find great comfort in their religious or spiritual beliefs. Is this something you identify with?'

- 'You know you have a choice about where you would like your end of life care to take place and I wonder if you would like to talk through these options.'
- 'There may be things you want to say to your family—or arrangements that need to be made. Have you thought about this and can we help in any way?'

Being too attached to one's own agenda can inhibit progress so remain aware of the potential to manipulate discussions by imposing one's own beliefs on to the patient. Instead help them identify and 'own' their emotions and decisions by allowing the communication to be patient-led. Develop strategies for 'walking alongside the patient' and use empathic phrases such as 'I sense this is difficult for you so just take your time' to reassure that you are working at their pace.

Responses to difficult questions

Patients often project on to staff their own fears around death and dying. 'I think I am dying' one seriously ill patient said. Paralysed with anxiety, the nurse replied jovially 'Well, we've all got to die sometime', which immediately inhibited further discussion and left the patient's needs unmet.

Whilst platitudes, such as 'no-one has said that to me', 'of course you're not', or 'don't say that; you never know what's round the corner', might address the discomfort of the nurse, they deny the patient the opportunity to verbalize innermost fears and feelings that could have been facilitated by interventions such as:

- 'What makes you think that'; or
- 'I'm aware that you have been having a difficult time lately but what's changed so significantly to make you think you are dying?'; or
- 'Do you think you are or feel you are?'

These interventions of empathic understanding make the patient feel they have been heard, their concerns recognized, and that they have been given permission to expand.

> And remember, when you don't have the words, a silent presence or a gentle touch is enough.

Silences in conversations are significant and often occur following shocking news or when the patient is required to deliberate and process new information. Normal convention dictates that silences should be broken because they are uncomfortable to tolerate but, in a therapeutic setting, silences often denote that the patient is undergoing a period of deep reflection as they reframe thoughts and questions. To interject too soon can inhibit further exploration on the part of the patient who then feels that permission to speak the 'unspeakable' has been denied because it is too painful for the listener to hear. Sometimes patients need help to re-enter the present and a sensitive way of appropriately moving on from a silence and getting back to the 'here and now' is to say 'I am noticing you are very quiet and wonder what you are thinking.'

Ending a discussion also needs sensitive handling. Patients need sufficient time to absorb what they have heard and to accommodate the accompanying emotions. It is imperative that the patient is left emotionally intact following any discussion, that all questions have been honestly answered, and, if distress is being experienced, there is someone available to offer support. This might be helped by summarizing what has been said, including an acknowledgement of the difficult things discussed, but with a definite person or point of contact for future questions, which often arise as soon as the doctor leaves.

Communicating with family members

> Poor communication leaves doctors and family members stressed and dissatisfied; it also has the potential to neglect the patient's wishes

We should be mindful of the needs of the nuclear family when dealing with patients who are facing end of life care and be sensitive to their issues.

On a practical level flexible visiting hours should be allowed and close family members should be invited to participate in some care tasks, which can make them feel useful rather than useless. Appropriate facilities should be made available such as a quiet room where they can reflect privately and express the thoughts and emotions that they find too painful to share with their dying loved one. See 'Integrated care pathway for end of life care', p. 252.

Families often need help to mourn the lost health of their loved one as they too dip in and out of the grieving process, and onward referral for emotional support may be appropriate. They may also need help on how to best relate to their dying loved one—how to behave around someone who is dying. Family adaptation to the demands imposed by the dying requires variations in ordinary social roles that can often create or increase tensions within interpersonal relationships. Medical staff should, wherever possible:

- meet with significant family members in a quiet, private setting with no distractions and a box of tissues handy to discuss diagnosis and future care plans;
- consider the timing of sharing bad news and ensure it is broken in a way that will minimize the distress the family will experience;
- ensure psychological support is available for the family at this time;
- allow sufficient time for questions;
- offer to meet with the family again and/or offer a time when you will be available for ongoing consultations;
- respect family members' knowledge of their loved one's illness and symptoms together with their management skills and ability to cope with the situation;
- respond positively to their desire that their loved one gets the best treatment available;
- recognize their anger which is sometimes displaced on to staff and 'hold' it;
- normalize the grief process;
- do not pass judgement when families find it too painful to manage the care of their loved one;
- work at their pace and keep them informed at all times;
- ensure they have access to information packs on what to do following a death and where bereavement support can be accessed.

And bear in mind that, after death, many relatives still have a need to remain in contact with the renal unit as it provides a way of remaining in touch with their loved one.

Communicating on issues around sexuality and intimacy

> We've been married over 20 years and, apart from when the kids were born, have never spent a night apart. I long to climb into that bed and just hold him

Sexuality continues to be important at end of life but is often not included in discussion with patients. Emotional connection to others is an integral component of sexuality taking precedence over physical expression. Lack of privacy, shared rooms, staff intrusion, and single beds are all considered barriers to expressing sexuality in hospital or hospice settings, but rarely are arrangements made for patients to share intimacies. Perhaps this is because it is assumed that sexual attraction and needs diminish with the progression of illness and, whilst this might be so, the need for 'closeness' would appear to be ever present. Patients should be asked how their distress could be minimized with interventions such as:

- 'It's quite difficult to have private moments in this setting isn't it, and I am aware that you are finding this upsetting. Can you think of anything we can do to improve things for you and your partner?'

Following which creative solutions should be sought to try and address unmet needs.

Communicating within teams and information sharing

Information sharing should occur both between multidisciplinary team members (with consideration given to the need for confidentiality) and also between patient and caregiver.

In palliative care, roles overlap and this can lead to blurred boundaries and uncertainty as to who does what. Staff need a strong sense of their own professional identity to allow others to share aspects of their work without feeling threatened.

Each professional needs to remember that they are part of a team with colleagues to support and be supported by. When in doubt or overwhelmed by sadness, seek this support. It is not a sign of weakness but an acknowledgement that we recognize our own areas of unmet need—that we too need to be cared for.

Multidisciplinary meetings (MDTs) are a good place to start and it is essential that each member's opinions and assessments are respected and valued and a 'named' person identified to carry out specific tasks. Conflicts do sometimes arise as the priority for reducing delayed discharges takes precedence over what might be in the patient's best interest, which is why it is imperative to include everyone involved in the patient's care in the decision-making—including the patient.

Good practice

- Elicit the views and assessments of everyone involved in the patient's care within the discussion and decision-making framework. This includes family members, nursing staff and other professionals, and, of course, the patient.
- Encourage sharing of thoughts, ideas, feelings. Sometimes creative thinking can benefit patient and carers. For instance, giving a patient day or weekend release with the appropriate level of support can provide opportunities to deal with unfinished business and goodbyes.
- Consistent communication is essential. Sometimes it is advisable for one named doctor or nurse to communicate with family members to reduce the possibility of mixed messages.
- Collaboration—not just within the renal team but with community teams, district nurses, social services, and GPs—will enhance end of life care.
- There should be a contemporaneous record of MDT discussions.

Collaborative working at its best utilizes the skills and expertise of each discipline as they work towards providing the highest level of care for their patient. Individuals should not assume they fully understand the role of another team member but, in order to appreciate them, should listen to shared information and knowledge. This will lead to effective working within a multidisciplinary team framework

An example of good practice

John had been in hospital for 7 weeks and was desperate to be discharged home. He lived with his two children aged 20 and 22 and his wife who had ongoing mental health problems. He had been deemed 'medically fit for discharge' but the family had raised concerns and a case discussion was called to evaluate the situation

- His children felt he would be unsafe at home and that his needs were too great to be met by a large package of care. But they had not felt able to discuss their concerns with their father as he had a history of bullying and making them feel as if they had failed him by not supporting his wish to be discharged home
- The doctors felt his prognosis was between 3–6 months and therefore referral for a hospice bed at this stage was not appropriate
- The OT spoke of the impossibility of providing ramps to access the property and other equipment that might have made discharge home a reality
- The social worker reported that the maximum number of calls that could be put in a day was four and that there was no night cover
- The CPN for the wife related that her client was at risk of an emotional breakdown if she had to participate in the care of her husband
- The multidisciplinary assessment indicated that John's needs could not be met within the home environment and that a nursing home placement should be sought
- The family was asked whether they wanted to discuss this with their father or whether they would prefer a member of the renal team to do so. They overwhelmingly supported the latter
- The team then explored who was best placed to broach the subject of a placement with John
- The social worker had not had any involvement with the patient—only with the family—and she was identified as the most appropriate person to continue supporting them during this transition
- The nursing staff felt John 'wouldn't listen' to them and would refuse to accept a placement
- However, one of the senior doctors related that he had a good relationship with the patient and felt he could help him accept that this really was the only option at this time
- The team had acknowledged that it was this gentleman's wish to return home; however, it was not felt to be a realistic or safe option.

John was discharged to a nursing home for placement and end of life care

Communication and team sharing can be improved by:
- learning about each other's roles through education, group discussion, and presentations;
- participation in advanced communication skills courses;
- use of clinical supervision;

- use of reflective practice;
- encouragement in full participation at MDTs;
- making sure everyone is heard;
- seeking feedback from patients, families, and other staff members on how a situation has been managed;
- learning from feedback or debriefing sessions;
- carrying out audits.

It is hugely rewarding to see positive outcomes that have arisen through effective communication, information sharing, and collaborative working. It is only by acknowledging and working with the different areas of expertise and specialist knowledge that team members bring that we will be able to provide the optimal level of patient care.

The place of supportive and palliative care in end-stage renal disease

Introduction and definitions

'You matter because you are you, and you matter to the end of your life'

Dame Cicely Saunders 1919–2005

The active total care of patients whose disease is not responsive to curative treatment. Control of pain, of other symptoms, and of psychological, social, and spiritual problems is paramount. The goal of palliative care is achievement of the best quality of life for patients and their families. Many aspects of palliative care are also applicable earlier in the course of the illness **in conjunction with conventional care for the renal patient**

Modified WHO 1990

The modified WHO definition of palliative care above contains the essence of supportive and palliative care. It can be applied equally to those with renal disease as to the cancer sufferers for whom it was originally written as it encompasses all domains of care, includes the family and carers, and recognizes the need for such care earlier in the disease than is frequently recognized currently for patients with ESRD. This type of care is sometimes separated into supportive care and palliative care, which are described below.

Supportive care
The National Council for Palliative Care (NCPC) defines supportive care as follows.

'Supportive care helps the patient and their family to cope with their condition and its treatment—from pre-diagnosis, through the process of diagnosis and treatment, to cure, continuing illness, or death and into bereavement. It helps the patient to maximize the benefits of treatment and to live as well as possible with the effects of the disease. It is given equal priority alongside diagnosis and treatment.'

Supportive care should be fully integrated with diagnosis and treatment. It is part of a team's overall service provision, and will be provided at times during a patient's illness as part of the patient's holistic care. Other specialists may be brought in for particular aspects of care.

The NCPC goes on to describe what it encompasses:
- self-help and support;
- user involvement;
- information giving;
- psychological support;
- symptom control;
- social support;
- rehabilitation;

- complementary therapies;
- spiritual support;
- end of life and bereavement care.

Providing supportive care for the patient is part of the renal team's holistic care of their patients; it is provided by different members of the team at different times. Other specialists and disciplines may be brought in when needed to contribute to that care.

Palliative care

This is defined by NICE as follows.

> Palliative care is the active holistic care of patients with advanced progressive illness. Management of pain and other symptoms and provision of psychological, social, and spiritual support is paramount. The goal of palliative care is achievement of the best quality of life for patients and their families. Many aspects of palliative care are also applicable earlier in the course of the illness in conjunction with other treatments

It aims to:
- affirm life and regard dying as a normal process;
- provide relief from pain and other distressing symptoms;
- integrate the psychological and spiritual aspects of patient care;
- offer a support system to help patients live as actively as possible until death;
- offer a support system to help the family cope during the patient's illness and in their own bereavement.

General palliative or supportive care is provided by all doctors and nurses who provide day to day care of patients. Specialist palliative care is provided by a multidisciplinary team who has specialized in it and who may practise within a specialist palliative care setting or in an advisory role either in hospital or the community.

Working alongside

Palliative care provides a philosophy of care that accompanies the patient whatever setting they are in. Specialist palliative care services are complementary to those of the renal team. Team members work alongside their renal colleagues, except for hospice in-patient end of life care, when care of the patient will be assumed by the palliative care team. In all other settings the two teams need to work in tandem, so the patient continues to receive the expertise of the renal multidisciplinary team plus the additional knowledge of specialist palliative care, thus providing the best possible care for the patient. When the patient is at home the primary care team will lead the patient's care but be able to utilize the expertise of either team as required

Why is palliative care needed?

The morbidity and mortality of patients with end-stage renal disease has been described in the preceding chapters. It is recognized that they experience the following.

- Multiple symptoms.
- Multiple losses:
  - employment;
  - role in family and at work;
  - appearance changes;
  - increasing dependence, which may lead to guilt;
  - sexual health;
  - financial.
- An incurable condition.
  - Even with a transplant previous morbidity may persist and antirejection drugs are lifelong and often have significant and even life-threatening side-effects.
- Relentlessly increasing comorbidity.
- Increasing dependence.

As more attention is paid to these aspects of the care of this group of patients so the importance of their supportive care during ongoing management and more intensive palliative care at times of crisis or as end of life approaches is recognized.

Provision of specialist palliative care services in UK

Specialist palliative care services are provided in a number of ways.

- Specialist in patient facilities either in hospice or hospital.
- Hospital advisory teams.
- Home support:
  - advisory teams working alongside GP and district nurse;
  - intensive home nursing or 'hospice at home' services for end of life care.
- Day hospice.
- Bereavement care.
- Education and training.

Most palliative care services will accept referrals of patients with ESRD, though not all may be able to accept patients into specialist palliative care beds, usually due to the relative shortage of these beds. A few voluntary organizations may only accept certain categories of patient, such as only cancer patients. This distinction is gradually being reduced as the needs of non-cancer patients are increasingly recognized.

Further information
http://www.ncpc.org.uk/palliative_care.html

Referral and joint working

Indications for referral to palliative care services

Many patients will not require referral to a palliative care service; rather they will receive palliative care from their renal and primary care teams. For some, the symptoms from their disease and its complications, or the severity of psychological, social, or spiritual issues may be sufficiently severe to require referral for help in their management. Other patients may request end of life care in a hospice or palliative care unit setting. Possible points in a patient's disease when specialist palliative care may enhance the care of the renal patient are listed below.

- Severe symptoms that are difficult to control and affecting quality of life.
- New significant diagnosis of a life-limiting illness while receiving renal replacement therapy.
- Increasing symptoms from comorbid conditions, such as:
  - diabetic neuropathy;
  - peripheral vascular disease;
  - arthritis.
- At the onset of conservative management:
  - in conjunction with renal and primary care team;
  - to ensure optimal symptom management.
- Falling performance status or other parameters identified in Chapter 8.
- Recognizing dying, which leads clinicians to believe prognosis less than a year.
- Patients who develop renal failure as a consequence of other life-threatening condition or its treatment, e.g. cancer.
- Around the decision to stop dialysis:
  - for psychological support;
  - symptom control;
  - family support;
  - help with planning re preferred place of care;
  - bereavement support.
- Terminal care—where there are difficult symptoms or complex psychological needs.

Joint working

There are many ways in which renal and palliative care teams can work together to improve patient care.

- Develop a supportive care group of renal and palliative care professionals to lead in improving care by initiatives such as:
  - guidelines for end of life care;
  - guidelines for symptom control;
  - use of integrated care pathway (ICP) for end of life care;
  - written information for primary care;
  - notification of conservative management decision on database;
  - written information for patients—choosing not to dialyse;
  - improved physical facilities for inpatients.

- Joint education programmes.
- Change ways of working by:
  - joint renal/palliative care clinics;
  - preparative discussions with community palliative care services;
  - integration of nursing and psychological assessment notes;
  - identification of key worker;
  - critical event debriefing;
  - use of advanced directives;
  - open door policy to support for bereaved family;
  - open culture in discussing death and dying during pre-dialysis meetings.

Ethical and legal considerations

Principles of ethical decisions

For most patients with end-stage renal disease decisions concerning current management and future care are made as part of an ongoing dialogue with their renal physician within a relationship that has built up over many years. Difficult decisions are then made on the basis of previous honest communication and trust. As the UK law stood until April 2007, if the patient later develops incapacity, the team, led by the consultant makes decisions regarding end of life care 'in the patient's best interest'. This ongoing relationship, which will include family members if present and other members of the renal multidisciplinary team, will contribute to the decision-making process. The overriding standard of care is to act in the patient's best interest. Guidance and information supporting ethical decision-making with respect to end of life care is found in the GMC document: *Withholding and withdrawing life-prolonging treatments: good practice in decision-making*.[1]

The key GMC principles are summarized as follows.

- Respect for human life and best interests.
  - The offering of treatments where benefits outweigh burdens must take all factors into consideration, including the fact that prolonging life, though usually so, might not always be in the patient's best interest if treatment, such as dialysis, proves excessively burdensome and therefore provides no net benefit.
- End of natural life.
  - Where life is coming to a natural end, doctors should not strive to prolong dying.
- Adult patients who can decide for themselves have the right to refuse treatment even where the decision results in harm or their own death.
- Adult patients who cannot decide for themselves have equal rights (see discussion below: Mental Capacity Act).
- Choosing between options, where there are differences of view about best interests:
  - these will be individual decisions;
  - there is no ethical or legal obligation on the doctor to provide treatment that is not clinically indicated;
  - where the patient lacks capacity it is important to take time to try to reach a consensus and it may be appropriate to seek a second opinion, or other independent or informal review (see below).
- Concerns about starting then stopping treatment.
  - It may be appropriate to initiate treatment that may be of some benefit while decisions are made or to allow the natural development of a situation.
  - It is important to be clear that a review of treatment will take place and that it may be withdrawn if ineffective or too burdensome.
- Artificial nutrition and hydration.
  - Not eating or drinking is part of the natural dying process.
- Non-discrimination.
- Care for the dying.
  - Communication with the patient can enable the dying patient to express their wishes.

- Care should be with the same respect and standards for all patients—see Chapter 12.
- Conscientious objections.
  - Where a decision is taken to withdraw treatment and a clinician has a conscientious objection to that decision they 'may withdraw from the care of that patient, while ensuring that arrangements have been made for another suitably qualified colleague to take over their role, so that the patient's care does not suffer.'
- Accountability.
  - 'Doctors are responsible to their patients and society at large, while being individually accountable to the GMC and in the courts for their decisions about withholding and withdrawing life-prolonging treatments.'

To put the principles into practice the GMC has produced a 'Good practice framework'.

Good practice framework Relevant key items are as follows.
- The clinical responsibility remains with the consultant.
- A thorough assessment of situation and prognosis with consultation with the whole renal team and seeking a second opinion if necessary should be undertaken.
- Options for treatment considering burdens and benefits will be weighed before reaching a decision.
- In an emergency where there is uncertainty about appropriateness of treatment then treatment may be initiated till there is time for a full review of the situation.
- The patient's views will be sought, providing them with sufficient information regarding diagnosis, prognosis, and burdens and benefits of treatment.
  - Where option to discuss stopping life-sustaining treatment is involved patients should have the option to discuss how they would like their care managed—see also 'Renal NSF' on the next page.
- Discussions should be handled sensitively and if necessary over several meetings, respecting a patient's decision not to take part in those discussions if they so wish.
- Where patients lack capacity and the patient's wishes are not known, the senior clinician has responsibility to make a decision about what course of action would be in the patient's best interests.
  - Guidance is in accordance with that described below under Mental Capacity Act 2005.
  - The aim should be to reach a consensus, enabling all relevant people to contribute but ultimately the responsibility lies with the consultant.
  - Where there is difficulty reaching a consensus, despite multidisciplinary clinical discussion, independent or ethical review should be considered, using legal advice where necessary.
- Decisions that will result in death must be communicated effectively to all members of the clinical team, in writing as well as verbally, ensuring also that patient and family wishes for end of life care are known—see Chapter 12.

- Decisions should be reviewed if clinical circumstances change or the patient does not progress as predicted.
- These decisions should be reviewed in team audit discussion to ensure continued learning to improve practice.

UK National Service Framework (NSF) for renal services: markers of good practice

The *UK National Service Framework for Renal Services, part 2: chronic kidney disease, acute renal failure and end of life care* was published in 2005.[2] It contains specific quality requirements around end of life care that, if followed, contribute to the ethical management of these patients.

Quality requirement 4 states that 'people with established renal failure receive timely evaluation of their prognosis, information about the choices available to them, and for those near the end of life a jointly agreed palliative care plan built round their individual needs and preferences'. The markers of good practice shown in the box contribute to decision-making and care of the patient and thus ethical end of life care.

Renal NSF, part 2. Markers of good practice

- Access to expertise in discussion of end of life issues
  - This emphasizes the importance of communication—see below
- Principles of shared decision-making. See also 'Guidelines from the Renal Physicians Association of the USA guideline' opposite
- Training in symptom relief relevant to this group of patients
  - This is key to good end of life care—see Chapters 6, 7, and 12
- Prognostic assessment based on available data available to all patients with stage 4 disease and beyond
  - Patients and families can only make informed choices if they know the possible outcomes from the particular actions under consideration
- Information about treatment choices
  - This includes non-dialytic therapy or stopping renal replacement therapy once started
- Jointly agreed care plan in line with palliative care principles
  - This will mean joint working with primary care and palliative care teams
- Ongoing medical care for those who choose not to dialyse
  - Patients are reassured to know that the no dialysis option is not a no treatment option but rather a maximal supportive care option with full medical care to maintain function as long as possible
- Support to die with dignity
  - It is beholden on the physician to ensure the quality of care is maintained to death and into bereavement
- Culturally appropriate bereavement support to family, carers, and staff
  - Failure to do this will impact on the care families and professional carers are able to provide.

Guidelines from the Renal Physicians Association of the USA

In the USA the recognition of the need for clinical practice guidelines in this area produced the Renal Physicians Association and the American Society of Nephrology clinical practice guideline (RPA/ASN guideline): shared decision-making in the appropriate initiation of and withdrawal from dialysis.[3]

The nine recommendations in this guideline, summarized in the box, form a framework for decision-making based on expert consensus opinion backed by systematic literature review where appropriate and based on US statutory law and ethical principles.

Guidelines from the Renal Physicians Association of the USA

- **Shared decision-making:** that is at minimum between patient and physician but may include wider renal team and family or friends with patient's consent
- **Informed consent or refusal.** Information to include diagnosis, prognosis, and all possible treatment options, including that of not starting dialysis
- **Estimating prognosis.** This is to inform decision-making and should take into account up to date prognostic data
- **Conflict resolution.** A systematic approach to decision-making should be made whether it is between the patient and the renal team or within the renal team
- **Advance directive.** Where one is in place it should be honoured, and renal physicians should encourage dialysis patients to consider making one
- **Withholding and withdrawing dialysis.** It will be appropriate to withhold or withdraw dialysis in certain situations
- **Special patient groups.** Those with a terminal illness other than renal failure or in whom vascular access is technically impossible
- **Time-limited trial of dialysis.** Uncommon in UK
- **Palliative care.** The ongoing care for those who decide not to dialyse, often referred to as supportive care in UK, or the care of those who stop dialysis

A process of ethical decision-making

Alvin Moss in *Supportive care for the renal patient* goes on to tabulate a process of ethical decision-making in patient care, similar to the GMC guidance but specific to withholding and withdrawing from dialysis, which includes steps for conflict resolution if present.[4] This is summarized and adapted slightly as follows.

● Identify the ethical question.
● Gather all medical and social facts.
● Identify relevant guidelines and values—particularly distinctive values for patient or family.
● Look for solution that respects guidelines and values to proceed on if solution not possible.
● Propose possible alternative solutions.
● Evaluate these against values identified.
● Identify the best option with justification for choice.

An illustrative case study

What happens when a patient does not have the capacity to make an informed decision and the wishes of the next of kin regarding treatment differ from those of the physician? The following case study sets out such a scenario.

A profoundly physically disabled patient with severe learning difficulties is being looked after in a care home. With impaired cognition and unable to speak, mobilize, or feed himself he develops end-stage kidney disease requiring renal replacement therapy. A clinical decision not to offer treatment was made based on the facts that:
● the patient could not give informed consent to a rigorous dialysis regime;
● that quality of life would not be enhanced by undergoing renal replacement therapy.
However, the next of kin has argued that the patient's quality of life, although limited, is worthy of life-sustaining treatment and a transplant from next of kin is requested

Can this difficult situation be helped by working through Alvin Moss's process of ethical decision-making?

1 Identify the ethical issue
The professional opinion of what is in the patient's best interest differs from that of the next of kin.

2 Gather all medical and social facts
In this case this was done by referring to a renal social worker to carry out an independent psychosocial assessment. This was achieved by seeing the patient in his home setting where he was participating in his routine daily activities.

It was determined if there were any absolute medical contraindications to proceeding.

3 Identify relevant guidelines and values, i.e. particularly distinctive values for that patient or family or, in this case, his carers

This visit enabled the social worker to gain insight into what was important to the patient, and to invite the opinions of staff who were involved in his daily care. It also afforded an opportunity to educate those staff about the practicalities of dialysis and to define their role in terms of his care if he became a renal patient. The staff were able to offer observations, from their knowledge of the patient, on issues around quality of life for this individual. They were also asked how they felt the patient would cope with the regime and whether they could provide the increased level of care that would be required in order to meet his needs if he embarked on renal replacement therapy. Family and carers wished to pursue renal replacement therapy after this meeting so they proceeded to the next step.

4 Look for a solution that respects guidelines and values

To proceed with this a multidisciplinary meeting (to include general practitioner, district nurse, nephrologist, care staff, social worker, dialysis sister, next of kin) was convened to discuss a plan of care and the logistics of implementation. Prior to this meeting practical hurdles such as the acceptance of blood tests were checked and it was agreed that dialysis would not be possible.

5 Propose possible alternative solutions

The possibility of a family donor transplant was considered. However, it was felt the case should go before an ethical committee for a decision. It was felt a disinterested opinion was desirable as the child could not consent and the next of kin was also the potential donor.

6 Evaluate these against values identified

Before this could be done, the child moved cities and care was transferred to another team. It was therefore not possible to proceed to the next step.

7 Identify the best option with justification for choice

References
1 http://www.gmc-uk.org/guidance/archive/library/witholding_and_withdrawing/witholding_lifeprolonging_guidance.asp
2 Department of Health (2005). The National Service framework for Renal Services. Part Two: Chronic Kidney Disease, Acute Renal Failure and End of Life Care. Department of Health.
3 Renal Physicians Association and American Society of Nephrology (2000). *Shared decision-making in the appropriate initiation of and withdrawal from dialysis*, Clinical Practice Guidelines number 2. RPA, Rockville, Maryland.
4 Moss A (2004). Introduction to ethical case analysis. In *Supportive care for the renal patient* (ed. EJ Chambers *et al.*), pp. xv–xix. Oxford University Press, Oxford.

Further information
Further ethical principles that guide this practice have been produced by the UK Ethics Clinical Network at *http://www.ethox.org.uk/Ethics/eendlife.htm*

Choosing conservative management of ESRD

When dialysis was first available it was limited to the fit under-50-year-old breadwinner. With technical advances and the increasing availability of renal replacement therapy there has been a continuing increase in uptake, which now includes the very elderly and those with multiple comorbidities. However, take-up, even in developed economies, is variable from 103 per million population (pmp) in the UK to 333 pmp in the US. Not all patients do well on dialysis and for some there is a marked deterioration in quality of life, though this is not entirely predictable.

> **Dialysis: factors associated with a poor prognosis**
>
> • Low Karnofsky performance status (KPS)
> • Multiple comorbidity
> • Frailty
> • Age > 75y

However, all nephrologists will know of patients in whom a poor outlook was predicted but who experience good quality of life on dialysis and vice versa.

Factors to consider before deciding to withhold or withdraw dialysis

Where possible, discussions around decisions about starting dialysis should be conducted before the absolute necessity to dialyse intervenes. This gives the patient and family time to assemble and assimilate the relevant information. This will also allow them to receive information from all members of the renal multidisciplinary team, sometimes in their own home. Some patients are helped in their decision-making by talking to current renal patients. Mailloux describes eight factors that should be considered before a decision to withhold or withdraw dialysis is made.[1]

• Assessment of the patient's decision-making capacity—see legal considerations and capacity.
• Assessment of possible reversible factors.
• Detailed and effective communication with the patient.
• Family involvement, with appointment of surrogate (in US and also in UK after April 2007: referred to as 'lasting power of attorney').
• Interdisciplinary dialysis team involvement.
• The presence of an advance directive, either through a living will (called 'advance decisions' in UK after April 2007) or health care proxy ('lasting power of attorney').
• A trial period of dialysis if appropriate.
• Commitment to support the patient's decision whether it is to continue to dialyse, withdraw, or forego initiation.

Assessment of possible reversible factors

Renal physicians will always wish to assure themselves and the patient and family that all possible interventions have taken place to optimize the patient's medical management, including the dialysis prescription and, where appropriate, social support. All reversible acute events will need to be addressed before considering a decision to withdraw, including an assessment for depression and, if in doubt, assessment of cognitive function and capacity.

Detailed and effective communication with the patient

As indicated, discussions to withhold dialysis should if possible take place over time and at the patient's pace. It will be important to ensure the patient has understood the consequence of a decision either to withhold dialysis or withdraw from it. Physicians should check their patient's understanding before a decision is agreed, and allow the patient access to any other professionals the patient may wish to consult and appropriate support or counselling to assist decision-making.

Family involvement, with appointment of surrogate

If possible, and with the patient's permission, it is important to keep families in the picture if a patient is considering not starting dialysis. At times a decision made over time between the physician and patient, perhaps with a family member present, is challenged strongly by another family member who has not been party to the early discussions. This can lead to considerable distress both for the patient and frequently for the team looking after the patient where the team believed a fully informed decision had been made and is now challenged often when time is short.

Sarge was a 50-year-old clinically obese diabetic with visual impairment, neuropathy, and CKD that required imminent dialysis. He was unable to mobilize and lived out his life in the confines of the family living room with his wife acting as his primary carer. Whilst he had made a fully informed decision to be conservatively managed, his family were opposed and urged him to have a trial period on dialysis before making a firm decision. He steadfastly refused, which caused enormous emotional pain, turmoil, and anger for his family who felt rejected and abandoned, feeling that, no matter how much they cared for him, no matter what they did for him, it simply wasn't enough for him to want to continue to live.

Interdisciplinary dialysis team involvement

It is important that the contributions of the whole renal team are taken into account, particularly where decisions are difficult, as non-medical team members may have unique insight into factors that do not emerge in the medical consultation. The usefulness of a multidisciplinary team meeting comes into play here. See also the box above.

The presence of an advance directive

In the event of the loss of capacity for decision-making, advance care planning with respect to refusal of treatment may help clinicians and family ascertain what those individuals' wishes were if the circumstances described in the advance directive apply to the clinical situation at the time. However, unless the advance directive is very detailed, it is likely that the specific clinical situation at the time may not be covered. Current and future UK law enshrines the principle of doing what is 'in the patient's best interest'. The difficulty may come in interpretation; an advance directive may help those making decisions when viewed in the light of previous communication and family knowledge of the individual. Use of Alvin Moss's suggested process for reaching decisions may help in the presence of uncertainty (see pp. 193–4).

A trial period of dialysis if appropriate

Formal trials of dialysis are uncommon in the UK, but may occur informally if dialysis is necessary to allow the full elucidation of the clinical situation. If a trial occurs it is important that key parameters for assessment of success or otherwise are identified and that patient and family understand that a review will take place in a defined time, at which time there will be discussion about the appropriateness of continuing dialysis. Not uncommonly, a decision for a trial of dialysis is made when a patient is wavering about conservative management. Too often, no review takes place after the 'trial' and the patient becomes committed to an extended time on dialysis.

Whole team commitment to support the patient and family's decision

When a decision has been made with appropriate consultation and discussion then it is important that the whole team commit to care based on that decision, even if some team members feel an unwise decision has been made.

Withdrawal from dialysis

Rates of withdrawal from dialysis are difficult to quantify as it varies markedly with age from around 6% of the under-60s to nearer 25% in the over-75s. In addition, it is not always listed as the cause of death or, conversely, may be listed when the patient dies after missing only one dialysis and actually dies from another condition. Much of the discussion above is equally relevant to decisions about withdrawal from dialysis. However, certain situations bring discussion about the option of stopping dialysis to the fore:

- rapid or clear reduction in performance status with increasing dependency;
- the development of severe symptoms from comorbid conditions;
- the development of other organ failure, particularly severe cardiac failure;
- the development of terminal malignancy;
- severe and symptomatic dementia;
- complications of peripheral vascular disease with multiple amputations.

Mailloux's factors need to be considered severally in these situations.

Additional considerations when withdrawing from dialysis
- Does the burden of treatment outweigh the benefit it provides?
- What is the patient's prognosis with and without treatment?
- Has the patient been assured of ongoing medical and nursing care, though with a change of emphasis to comfort and relief of symptoms?
- Have the patient and family had time to consider this decision?
- If the patient wishes, have they been informed of the nature of dying should they stop dialysis to balance in their judgement against the nature of likely events if they continue with dialysis? See also Chapter 12.

Reference

1 Mailloux LU (2004). Initiation and withdrawal of dialysis. In *Supportive care for the renal patient* (ed. EJ Chambers *et al.*), pp. 221–30. Oxford University Press, Oxford.

Renal replacement therapy and the elderly

Older patients are less likely to have a primary renal disease such as glomerulonephritis or polycystic kidneys and are more likely to have renal failure related to vascular or other comorbidities. They have other problems including impaired vision, deafness, poor mobility, arthritis, and cognitive problems. In addition, they are often socially isolated, may well have financial problems, and are often depressed due to loss of independence or bereavement. These factors are all problematic for any dialysis modality.

- For HD, the associated vascular disease leads to a high risk of failure for vascular access. This results in increased reliance on venous access with all the associated risks of infection. Failure of vascular access can necessitate frequent hospital admissions for often unpleasant and painful radiological and surgical procedures. Cardiac disease in these patients can also cause hypotension and arrhythmias while on HD.
- Peritoneal dialysis (PD) is a home-based treatment and causes less cardiovascular stress. Many elderly patients, however, cannot do this independently and would have to be dependent on carers.

Truth telling and collusion

A frequently discussed moral dilemma is whether or not a patient should be told the truth that they are dying—particularly if they haven't specifically asked to know their prognosis or if their family wishes to 'protect' them from the truth. Lies and half truths might be more comfortable for the informant but do the recipient a great disservice. Not being honest can induce short-lived euphoria, which can leave the patient feeling cheated when they learn the severity of their illness. By being economical or avoidant with the truth, we deny patients the right to make fully informed decisions about their future care and preferred place of death.

Professional carers must remember that they have a duty to the patient and, while supporting the relatives, must not withhold information from the patient at a relative's request unless the patient has explicitly stated that they wish for information to be given to their relative in preference to themselves. At the same time, the professional will not force unwanted information on a patient but rather check with them at each step of the information-giving when imparting bad news to ensure information is given at an appropriate pace for the individual. It helps to have explained to both relative and patient that no one will lie to them and, where possible, to impart bad news with the relative present.

If a patient asks if he is dying, he should receive an honest response followed by an invitation to seek further information as well as an opportunity to discuss future care options. Patients who appear not ready to hear the truth, could be gently asked: 'Shall I come back later, after you've had time to take in what's been said as we do need to discuss how you want to be looked after during the next weeks or months?'

Legal considerations: consent and capacity

Many end of life decisions depend on the patient understanding the nature of the possibilities open to him and the consequences of any decision to forego or stop treatment. Where there is doubt as to a person's capacity to make such decisions, their competence should be assessed. The law in England and Wales has changed and the effect of this will be described below

Patients who lack capacity

As the law stood in the UK in 2006, if a patient lacked capacity to make health-related decisions, particularly those relating to the withdrawal of a life-saving treatment, decisions were made by the healthcare team in the patient's best interest. Families should be involved in such decisions and would contribute to that decision-making through their prior knowledge of the patient. However, the final decision rested with the healthcare team, a fact that most next of kin are more comfortable with rather than finding themselves in the position of making life or death decisions themselves. Often being asked 'What do you imagine your father would have said if I had asked him whether he wanted to be resuscitated?' alleviates the burden and responsibility of decision-making and helps the healthcare team.

The law in the UK changed in 2007.

Mental Capacity Act 2005 (England)

The Mental Capacity Act provides a statutory framework to empower and protect vulnerable people who may not be able to make all of their own decisions. It sets out who can take decisions, in which situations, and how they should go about this. It relates to anyone lacking mental capacity, including a temporary loss of capacity. It will become a criminal offence of neglect to wilfully ill treat or neglect someone who lacks mental capacity. It comes into force during 2007 and applies to England and Wales; there is separate legislation in Scotland, The Adults with Incapacity (Scotland) Act 2000. It covers decisions of personal welfare including financial, social, and health aspects and introduces the role of 'lasting power of attorney', which replaces the previous 'enduring power of attorney'. Table 11.1 compares the legal considerations prior to and after implementation of the Act.

The aims of the 2005 Act are:
- better protection of the public;
- greater empowerment of patients;
- to clarify legal uncertainties.

Table 11.1 Comparison of the legal situation before and after the implementation of the Mental Capacity Act 2005

Domain	Pre Act 'enduring power of attorney' (EPA)	Post Act 'lasting power of attorney' (LPA)
Financial	Yes	Yes
Property	Yes	Yes
Health	No	Yes
Advanced refusal of treatment	No	Yes
Proxy health care decisions	No	Yes
Court of protection role	No	Yes
Assessment of capacity	Specialist—lawyer	Each healthcare professional
Decision in patient's best interest	Yes	Yes
Context for consideration of capacity	In the context of decisions with grave outcomes	In the context of every decision
New public body	Public guardianship office	Public guardian (registering authority for LPA & deputies)
Court of protection	No jurisdiction	Will have jurisdiction in relation to the Mental Capacity Act

Principles enshrined in the Act

- Assumption of capacity until proved otherwise.
- Individual not to be treated as being unable to make a decision unless all practicable steps to help them to do so have been taken without success.
- A person not to be treated as lacking capacity just because they make an unwise decision.
- Acts done or decisions made for someone must be in their best interest.
- Before an act is done or decision made consideration must be given as to whether the purpose for which it is needed could be achieved in a way less restrictive on the person's rights and freedoms of action.

Assumption of capacity and supported decision-making

The act sets out an assumption of capacity. It makes it clear that the professional:

- has an obligation to take all practical steps to help the person take his or her own decision;

- must make it clear that a person's age, appearance, condition, or behaviour does not by itself establish a lack of mental capacity;
- must give information in a way that is clear and easy to understand;
- must help the person who lacks capacity to communicate.

Each capacity assessment is decision-specific A person may have capacity to make some decisions but not others; at all times the person's best interest is the key principle governing all decision-making.

Defining mental incapacity

A person is deemed to have incapacity if they are unable to:
- understand the relevant information;
- retain that information sufficiently long to make a decision;
- use or weigh the information provided to make the decision;
- communicate their view on the decision they have made.

Determining a person's best interests
This is the same as current common law and should be done in two stages.
1 Consider all relevant circumstances through taking into account the following, which will help define best interests.
   - Involvement of the person who lacks capacity.
   - Having regard to the person's past and present wishes and feelings.
   - Consulting with others involved in the care of the person.
   - Excluding any discrimination.
2 Take the following steps.
   - Give consideration as to whether the person may have capacity in the future.
   - As far as possible, permit and encourage the person to participate in the decision-making.
   - Where a life-sustaining treatment such as dialysis is concerned, the person making the decision must not be motivated by a desire to bring about the person's death.
   - Consider where possible:
     — the person's previous wishes and feeling, beliefs, and values;
     — any other factor the person was likely to have taken into account.
   - Where practical take into account the views of anyone named by the person as someone to be consulted.

How the Act helps planning ahead for the renal patient
The Act can be used to help forward planning through more clearly defined means such as the following.
- The provision of lasting power of attorney, with a role in health as well as financial concerns.
- The use of advance decisions to refuse treatment, e.g. not wishing for dialysis.

- Enabling patients to make their wishes and feelings known:
  - patients should be encouraged to let professionals and family know what their wishes and feelings are;
  - there is no formal process but written statements given to professionals or recorded by them, while not legally binding, would be taken into consideration when considering a patient's best interest should they later lose capacity.

Further reading

The National Council for Palliative Care (2005). *Guidance on The Mental Capacity Act 2005.* NCPC Publications London UK.
http://www.dca.gov.uk/legal-policy/mental-capacity/index.htm

Lasting power of attorney and court-appointed deputies

Lasting power of attorney (LPA)
- This enables the patient to appoint someone they know and trust to make decisions for them.
- The areas covered by the Act include:
  - property and affairs, which replaces the former enduring power of attorney;
  - personal welfare, which is a new way to appoint someone to make health and welfare decisions;
  - specified matters relating to the person's welfare or property.
- They must be appointed when the person has capacity.
- They must be registered with the public guardian if the person loses capacity.
- The person chosen can only make decisions in the patient's best interest.
- An LPA in relation to welfare only applies if the person lacks capacity.

- An LPA for welfare can extend to giving or refusing consent to carry out or continue treatment but can only extend to life-sustaining treatment (such as dialysis) if expressly contained in the LPA and in writing and witnessed.

- The person appointing an LPA can appoint more than one holder.
- If doctors have any doubt about the validity or applicability of an advance decision they can provide treatment.

Court-appointed deputies (CADs)
CADs can be appointed by the court to make decisions on the patient's behalf without having to go back to the court and might be appointed in the following circumstances.
- Where there is a history of acrimony.
- Where it is in the patient's best interest to have deputy consult with all relevant people and have final authority.
- Exceptionally, if it is felt the patient is at risk of harm from family members.
- When there are a number of linked decisions that might otherwise each have to go back to court.

Advance decisions to refuse treatment

An advance decision to refuse treatment must relate to a specific treatment in specific circumstances.
- If it relates to a life-sustaining treatment such as dialysis it *must* be in writing, signed, and witnessed.
- It must also be valid and applicable.

Until the Act advance decisions to refuse treatment were regarded in a similar light to those that are usually spoken of as 'advance directives' or 'living wills'. The Act distinguishes between advance decisions to refuse treatment and those to request treatment—both are advance decisions, however.

- It is only an advance decision to refuse treatment that is applicable within the meaning of the Act and is therefore binding under the Act.

- It allows a person to refuse a particular treatment in advance.
- Is legally binding without the Act, but the Act provides greater safeguards.
- The decision must be made when the patient has capacity and only comes into force if the person develops a lack of capacity.
- Doctors can, however, provide treatment if they have any doubt about the validity of the advance decision.
- Patients may make non-binding written 'advance statements' about the sort of health care they would like to receive.
  - An 'advance decision' could be referred to as a 'binding advance decision to refuse treatment'.
  - An 'advance statement' is any other advance decision, not legally binding under the Act, but which must be taken into account when assessing a person's best interest.
- An advance decision is not valid if:
  - the patient has withdrawn it (must be in writing);
  - the patient has subsequently created an LPA who has authority to consent or refuse treatment;
  - the patient has done anything else inconsistent with the advance decision.
- An advance decision is *not* applicable if:
  - when the time comes to implement it the patient has capacity for that decision;
  - the treatment in question is not that stated in the advance decision;
  - any circumstances specified in the advance decision are absent;
  - there are reasonable grounds to think that the circumstances that currently prevail were not anticipated by the patient and if they had it might have affected their decision.

Communicating with patients about advance decisions

Communication regarding advance care decisions may not be easy to initiate, but giving in to feelings of discomfort and not broaching the subject may lead to outcomes not desired by the patient such as unwanted continuation of dialysis. Timely intervention is important and needs to be sensitively managed. If the question of resuscitation has not been discussed it might be introduced:

• 'We've discussed the progression of your illness and end of life preferences, but what we haven't touched on is how active you want us to be should your heart stop beating. Would you, for example, want us to attempt resuscitation?'

This could be accompanied by a description of the medical interventions that take place during this procedure and the likely outcomes.

What happens to the patient who loses capacity?

If there is no LPA or advance decision to refuse treatment, the patient will still be provided with care. Treatment decisions will be made in the patient's best interest by following the principles of the Act above, and decisions about withdrawal of life-sustaining treatment will be made in the same way as prior to the Act. Further possible resources include:

• an application to the court of protection for orders of the court in complex or difficult welfare decisions or one-off financial decisions or court-appointed deputies when a series of decisions are needed and a single application is insufficient;

• the appointment of an Independent Mental Capacity Advocate (IMCA) where the person has no next of kin and when decisions are being made about serious medical treatments. The withholding or withdrawing from dialysis would come in this category.

Multicultural issues

When English is not the patient's main language

There are occasions when non-English speaking patients need to make decisions about cessation of dialysis or advanced care directives. In this situation it is advisable to enlist the help of an interpreter rather than use a family member. Family members may interpret rather than translate, answering on behalf of the patient while thinking they know the right answer, or may indeed provide an answer that is contrary to the wishes of the patient.

By using an independent interpreter, you can be assured that the wishes of the patient are being accurately reflected (see box below).

Mr YS who was Chinese and 78 years old was a nursing home resident receiving thrice weekly HD. He was admitted to hospital with septicaemia. He had multiple comorbidities and a poor performance status. His command of English was poor and his family usually interpreted.

A palliative care team referral was made to help with symptoms of pain and distress.

Day 3 of admission
- One son wanted him to stop dialysis.
- Second son wanted him to continue.
- Inconsistent report of patient's view in the notes.
- Medical descriptors in the notes recorded that he was:
  - fed up;
  - upset;
  - refusing medication but not dialysis.

First interview on day 4 of admission
Patient was interviewed with second son present. It was recorded that the patient was:
- happy with quality of life;
- wanted to continue dialysis.

Second interview on day 5 of admission
Patient interviewed by an independent interpreter, a senior doctor, who recorded that patient was:
- alert and competent;
- clear that he wanted to stop dialysis.

Outcome
Patient therefore stopped dialysis. His notes record:
- demeanour changed—'settled, comfortable';
- pain more easy to manage for remainder of life.

He died on day 12. The staff caring for him had not felt that the unspoken language of the patient accorded with the second son's interpretation, and his body language after the decision to stop dialysis was made indicated concordance with what was happening to him

Attitudes to death in different cultures
It should also be remembered that diverse cultures have differing attitudes towards death and it might not be appropriate to talk about advance directives with a patient who believes discussions around death will hasten their demise. If unsure, it is better to ask the patient or family if it is all right to discuss these issues before embarking on such a discussion. At all times one must respect cultural beliefs and values and find a way of working with those that are not one's own.

The Assisted Dying for the Terminally Ill Bill 2005 (failed)

In 2006 Lord Joffe's new bill for assisted dying for the terminally ill received its second reading in the House of Lords. It was defeated, but it is likely there will be further attempts to make it law. The majority of doctors who voted from the Royal Colleges of Physicians, Radiologists, and General Practitioners and the Association of Palliative Medicine were against the bill. Key aspects of the bill were the following.

- A doctor may assist suicide for someone who is terminally ill and experiencing 'unbearable suffering' by the provision of medication.
- A terminal illness is defined as an inevitably progressive illness that is likely to result in death within 6 months.
- The patient must have been attended by a palliative care specialist to discuss the option of palliative care.
- If there is doubt about the patient's capacity they must be referred to a psychiatrist or psychologist to determine that they are not suffering from a disorder leading to mental impairment.
- No professional of any discipline is under any duty to participate in diagnosis, treatment, or other action authorized by the Act to which they have a conscientious objection.

A major concern to palliative care physicians is the assumption that one consultation with a palliative care professional constitutes 'palliative care'. As defined fully in Chapter 10, the provision of palliative care is a multi-disciplinary ongoing intervention that cannot be encapsulated in one meeting, nor can it be expected to achieve its full potential in that time.

- Current law prohibits a doctor from assisting a patient's suicide or deliberately killing a patient even after an explicit request by that patient
- Stopping dialysis is neither euthanasia nor assisted suicide but rather, when withdrawn in the presence of other progressive irreversible medical conditions, the withdrawal of futile treatment

End of life care

Introduction

Though recognizing the dying phase in patients with ESRD can be difficult (see Chapter 8), for those who withdraw from dialysis there is usually a predictable timescale to death. For some ESRD patients, where death is likely but not completely predictable, there can be preparation through consistently good symptom control and supportive care for the patient and family. These should be practised in conjunction with open and honest communication about likely prognosis throughout the course of the illness. This becomes particularly important as complications increase, often an indication that death is likely within months rather than years. Thus, if and when death occurs, opportunities for communication with those important to the patient have not been lost and attention to improved quality of life has been given.

Care at the end of life is as important and active as the care has been throughout the management of the renal disease. There is nonetheless a change in emphasis from prolongation of life and prevention of long-term complications to:

- relief of symptoms;
- maintenance of comfort;
- attention to psychological concerns of patient and family;
- consideration of spiritual needs (see Chapter 13);
- awareness of religious requirements (see Chapter 13).

Key issues to consider before cessation of dialysis

The exclusion of reversible factors Renal teams will have ensured all possible reversible causes of deterioration have been excluded or managed optimally and that, despite this, the current condition is seen as irreversible.

Effective communication with patient and family At all times contemporaneously documented communication between the professional carers and patient and family is essential for efficient team working and for the patient and family to have confidence in the team. A lack of effective means of communicating can lead to patients and their families receiving mixed messages about the plan and goals for care. A well documented plan will prevent this.

Decision-making capacity At the time of the decision-making the renal team will need to ensure that the patient has decision-making capacity with full understanding of the consequences of their decision. If capacity is lacking, the decision rests with the team led by the consultant, the most important factor in that decision being that any treatment should be in the patient's best interest. It is most likely, however, that the considerations of the family will hold significant weight in any decision and that renal teams will have had extensive discussions with them.

The Mental Capacity Act 2005 (comes into effect in 2007) determines that those with lasting power of attorney for their relation or who have been appointed as health proxy have the legal right to make decisions about treatment refusal, though not life-sustaining treatment such as dialysis, unless this has been specifically stated in writing and witnessed. (See Chapter 11.)

Advance care planning Advance care planning is a process that enables patients to document and communicate their views about appropriate future medical care when and if they become unable to make their own decisions and communicate them. With the passing of the Mental Capacity Act it is now possible for a patient to nominate a healthcare proxy to act as surrogate decision maker in the event of incapacity. Their opinion will contribute to decision-making. Advance decisions that are legally binding can only be made with respect of treatments that the patient wishes to refuse and the Act will not mean that unreasonable or inappropriate treatments can be demanded. (See Chapter 11.)

Multiprofessional team communication Information sharing must occur between multidisciplinary team members as well as between patient and caregiver, although issues around confidentiality have to be respected and sensitive information passed on only on a 'need to know' basis. It is helpful if there are formal means of communicating, such as multidisciplinary team meetings and handover sessions, as well as the informal verbal passing on of information. The use of one set of multidisciplinary notes for hospital inpatients also contributes to good communication.

Family/significant other involvement

'I live in Portsmouth and work full time. I really need to know the situation regarding my sister. If I need to be with her, then I need to organize my work and my family and it would help if I knew how long we were talking about'.

Appreciation of the physical, emotional, and economic demands that are placed upon families, friends, and carers during the terminal/end of life phase is essential. Even as they attend to the needs of their dying loved one, families and care-givers must continue to meet their current daily responsibilities towards work, their own families, and existing commitments. Carer fatigue, emotional distress, and economic pressure need to be acknowledged and appropriate levels of support and advice given. If prognostic timeframes can be given, it can put an uncertain future into perspective and facilitate immediate decision-making on the part of family members who are so often trying to organize their disorganized and disconnected lives in order to meet the needs of their loved one. If this proves impossible, you could say 'It is difficult to give accurate timeframes for patients such as your father, but I would estimate it could be…' Although uncertainty complicates decision-making, patients and families do appreciate an honest approach.

Whole team commitment to support patient and family whatever the decision

Teams may find it hard sometimes to accept a rational patient's decision to stop dialysis as some patients make a conscious decision to withdraw from treatment, whilst others are asked to support a clinical decision to withdraw. This can be a highly emotive situation where both family and patient are left in need of ongoing emotional support and it is crucial that staff are seen to work together and support the decision. (See the case study on p. 220.)

Informed consent to withdrawal of life-sustaining treatment should include honest, caring, and culturally sensitive communication with patients and family members. What we perceive to be a poor quality of life on dialysis might be considered a worthwhile existence to others. A glimpse of the patient's 'inner world' is gained not only through asking the right questions and actively listening to the answers, but by observing body language, heeding the tone of voice, understanding the patient's frame of reference and belief systems, and by noting what hasn't been said—what has so often been studiously avoided.

Case study

Michelle was 36 years old and a diabetic since the age of 12. Kidney failure came as a shock when diagnosed a year ago but she appeared to adapt well to PD and still managed to ride her horse and work part time. However, laser surgery on her eyes was unsuccessful and, within the space of just a few weeks, she had completely lost her vision. Unable to manage PD, she converted to HD and 3 months later asked to be withdrawn from treatment on the grounds that she couldn't tolerate the treatment and 'life was no longer worth living'. Exploration revealed that loss of vision and increased dependency were the main reasons for her reaching this decision.

Michelle never waivered from her wish to withdraw from treatment despite intense initial opposition from her husband and parents. Her end of life care was successfully managed in her own home, which is where she had requested to die. Team commitment to support her decision was crucial in facilitating her preferred place of care.

Further reading

Mailloux LU (2004). Initiation and withdrawal of dialysis. In *Supportive care for the renal patient*, (ed. EJ Chambers *et al.*), pp. 221–30. Oxford University Press, Oxford.

Where death is expected

Preparation for the dying phase should be made for this group of patients with consideration of the domains of care outlined on pp. 226–7. Each patient (or family in the case of someone who lacks competency) should be able to draw up and agree their own plan of care taking into account their wishes and their practical needs. It will not always be possible to accede to every wish, where lack of resources precludes either care at home or entry to a hospice if desired. However, every attempt should be made to provide the patient with an appropriate environment and dignity within the care facilities available and to enable those close to him or her to be present if that is his or her wish

Withdrawal or cessation of dialysis
- 10–25% of patients on dialysis choose to withdraw from it.
- The percentage increases with increasing age.
- Prognosis is short; median survival = 8 days (range 5–300 days).

Conservative management
- Around 10–20% of patients reaching ESRD will opt for maximal medical care but without dialysis.
- Prognosis variable, though usually measured in months, but may stretch to a year or more.
- Many die with rather than from their renal disease, however.
- One-third will die of uraemia.
- One-quarter will die of cardiac failure or pulmonary oedema, directly or indirectly related to their renal failure.

Failure of other vital organs
- Heart or liver but without explicit cessation of dialysis.
- Cardiovascular disease.
- Peripheral vascular disease.

Death from malignancy while continuing to dialyse
- Patients with a terminal malignant condition may choose to continue dialysis till their death is caused by the malignant condition rather than precipitate their certain death by stopping dialysis. Others use cessation of dialysis as a means of control of time of death.

DS had adult polycystic kidney syndrome, as did his brother who had died as a consequence. DS had received outpatient haemodialysis for many years when, at the age of 58, he developed a localized non-small-cell lung cancer that was treated with resection. He remained well for 18 months following this till he developed a biopsy-proven recurrence and over the next 18 months received three short courses of palliative radiotherapy to lymph node spread. Over the following 6 months symptoms from advancing cancer—hoarse voice, reducing performance status, and pain—developed till it was clear he was dying. As he approached his death he acknowledged and accepted that he was dying from his lung cancer and, when finally bedbound in hospital, was prepared to die from it but not from kidney failure insisting on dialysis to the end of his life

Terry was receiving chemotherapy for stage IV lymphoma when he went into renal failure. Depressed, scared, and aware that his prognosis was poor, he nevertheless elected to have dialysis. When asked why he had made this decision, he said 'I know if I don't have dialysis, I shall be dead within days or a couple of weeks and I don't think I can live every day just waiting for it to happen and wondering if I am going to wake up in the morning. It's a terrifying prospect—for me and my family—and I owe it to them to give it my best shot. You realize just how precious life is when you face death'

Technical difficulties with dialysis
- Lack of vascular access.
- PD often not possible.

Patient unable to cooperate or to tolerate dialysis
Refusal of dialysis in the non-competent patient leads to difficult ethical considerations and considerable stress to the team caring for the patient. Physical coercion may be considered assault. However, consideration of the patient's best interest may require you to attempt to continue dialysis, particularly if, as far as you can judge, that is what the patient had indicated that they would want in the given situation before loss of competence. (See Chapter 11.)

Quality in end of life care

Each of us will have our own view on what constitutes quality of care at the end of our lives and, though there will be differences between individuals, there are many common themes. Studies that help to guide us in identifying key domains and theme include work by PA Singer centred on the patients' perceptions of their own needs and wishes.[1] 48 dialysis patients were included in the group he questioned; they identified five domains of care that were important. If these are used as a guide to assessment alongside an approach that enables the patient to identify their own particular priorities, then it is likely that a personal plan of end of life care can be formulated that can enhance the care given to the patient and their family and the quality of the time left to that person. Additional resources include the London-based Age Concern report highlighting 12 principles of a good death as defined by its members (see box opposite).

Domains of end of life care[1]

- Receiving adequate pain and symptom management.
- Avoidance of inappropriate prolongation of dying.
- Achieving a sense of control.
- Relieving the burden to loved ones.
- Strengthening relationships with loved ones.

It behoves us to bear these domains in mind as we help patients and families prepare for death and to use them as a framework for assessment and planning care.

Last days of life

Recognizing the terminal phase

This is easy for those who choose to stop dialysis but much less clear for most ESRD patients, such as those dying from cerebrovascular disease or infection, for whom the dying phase is often not well defined. Sudden death is also common in ESRD and preparation for this can be achieved through good symptom management throughout illness and honest information about possible outcomes if the patient wishes. Supportive care as described above applies to these patients as well as those dying from their comorbid conditions or complications of chronic renal disease. See also Chapter 6.

An integrated care pathway for end of life care

The use of an integrated care pathway for end of life care. an initiative from Ellershaw and colleagues in Liverpool, is one way of supporting good practice at the end of life through prompts, guidelines, and documentation. This is described on p. 252.

Principles of a good death (from Age Concern UK)[2]

- To know when death is coming, and to understand what can be expected
- To be able to retain control of what happens
- To be afforded dignity and privacy
- To have control over pain relief and other symptom control
- To have access to information and expertise of whatever kind is necessary
- To have access to any spiritual or emotional support required
- To have access to hospice care in any location, not only in hospital
- To have control over who is present and who shares the end
- To be able to issue advance directives that ensure wishes are respected
- To have time to say goodbye, and control over aspects of timing
- To be able to leave when it is time to go and not to have life-prolonging treatment

References

1 Singer PA, Martin DK, Merrijoy K (1999). Quality end of life care: patients' perspectives. *J Am Med Assoc* **281** (2), 63–8.
2 Debate of the Age, Health and Care Study Group (1999). *The future of health and care for older people: the best is yet to come.* Age Concern, London.

Domains of care

Communication This is an ongoing process from the first meeting with the renal team. It is important that patients have the opportunity to learn of all options available to them, including that of stopping dialysis, in a supportive environment with time to ask questions. It is important for significant family members to be involved if the patient wishes. (See also Chapter 9.)

Comfort Practical ways to provide comfort include:
- stopping all unnecessary investigations;
- stopping routine monitoring, e.g. blood tests;
- rationalizing medication;
- a change in emphasis of nursing care from observation of BP/temperature, etc. to mouth care, pressure area care, and overall well-being.

Anticipatory prescribing for all pain and other symptoms

Crucial to relief of symptoms is the ready availability of the appropriate drug, correctly prescribed, so that there is no delay in patients obtaining attention to their symptoms. This is a key component of the Liverpool end of life care pathway and the following core symptoms should be addressed (see end of life symptom control guidelines pp. 242–5):
- pain;
- dyspnoea;
- agitation;
- retained respiratory secretions;
- fluid overload;
- nausea and vomiting.

Psychological

By the time many patients come to stop dialysis, they may have worked through the stages of grief as they approach death so that the stopping of dialysis is the final 'letting go'. Even for these people, however, there may be sadness and deep grief at the prospect of leaving their loved ones balanced by relief that they need struggle no longer. Fear of the unknown may still occur and, if time and cognition allow, active listening by staff and gentle reassurance that they will not be abandoned and will be cared for until the end are important. For others, deep-seated fears, inability to resolve longstanding family issues, or a lifetime of denial of the reality of their illness may lead to intense psychological distress at the end of life. Ideally, this would have been identified prior to the terminal phase when there might have been time for psychological support from a counsellor or psychologist. Even at this late stage, it is possible to help patients through open questions to elicit concerns. This gives the patient 'permission' to talk about what is troubling them most and listening in this context can be the most important intervention.

Social

Many patients have complex social concerns, such as care of a dependent relative, difficult financial concerns, and many others, that need the professional advice and support of a social worker and, if not resolved, act as a bar to peace at the end of life. All patients should be offered social support as should their carers. The carers may be struggling financially through the patient's illness with, for example, travel to hospital or loss of income. There may be other concerns such as dependent relatives at the same time as dealing with their own grief.

> LX, a 49-year-old single mother of two sons in their twenties, had sclerosing peritonitis after 8 years of PD. Prior to this, socially, her life had been extremely complex. One son, M, had been in prison for grievous bodily harm and the other was in prison for attempting to murder her. This son, K, also had a diagnosis of schizophrenia. M could not accept LX's ongoing support to K and, until her serious illness with peritonitis, had distanced himself from her. However, after she recovered and managed to convert to HD, he took her into his home to care for her. This was not entirely successful but, before she could make arrangements for herself elsewhere, the peritonitis flared up and she was re-admitted to hospital. She continued to deteriorate, and was showing signs of extreme anxiety that could not be resolved until she had honest answers about her prognosis, facilitated by her social worker. She was then able to explain her deep concerns that her sons might harm each other, and the social worker was able to enlist the help of another family member to bring about a reconciliation between the brothers with their mother days before she died.

Spiritual support

At no time in our lives are the questions concerning our very existence more important than when we face death. How we see ourselves in the scheme of things will influence profoundly how we feel at the end of our lives. Some patients will also have religious beliefs and practices that need attending to (see Chapter 13), but all will have their own spirituality even if not recognized and articulated as such. Hospitals, communities, nursing homes, and hospices all have access to spiritual advisors or carers. All patients should have their spiritual needs assessed and support offered. If the word spiritual is difficult to understand or a bar to opening a discussion, then talking of pastoral support sometimes helps unlock the door to communication about deep and troubling issues. Allowing the patient to tell his or her personal story gives them a sense of self-worth. The telling of the narrative of 'your' story turns a patient with ESRD into a person with a whole life and history behind them and a network of family and friends who will come after them. This listening endorses the person's self-worth and may help enable them to accept with a greater sense of peace distressing past events or family problems that had been causing anguish.

Symptoms at end of life

It is often suggested that if one had to choose a mode of death that was not sudden then dying of renal failure would be many clinicians' choice. This suggests a lack of recognition of the incidence and severity of renal-specific symptoms that occur in those who have chronic renal failure compared with those whose kidneys fail as a terminal event after previously normal or near normal renal function

Causes

The causes of different symptoms can classified as follows.

- Generic (possible whatever the cause of death). Likely to occur in some patients whatever cause of death and include:
  - pain, restlessness and agitation, nausea with or without vomiting, dyspnoea, and retained respiratory secretions.
- More likely in renal patients because of high incidence of comorbid conditions, e.g.
  - diabetic neuropathy;
  - peripheral vascular disease;
  - joint and bone disease.
- More likely in renal patients because of deteriorating renal function:
  - fluid overload;
  - uraemia and electrolyte disturbance;
  - acidosis;
  - neurological dysfunction.
- Renal-specific:
  - pain and ulceration caused by calciphylaxis;
  - adult polycystic kidney and liver pain;
  - amyloid deposition in joints.

Types of symptoms

The types of symptoms experienced include the following.

- Generic (* indicates symptoms likely to show increased incidence in ESRD):
  - pain;
  - dyspnoea*;
  - agitation and restlessness*;
  - retained respiratory secretions (death rattle)*;
  - nausea and vomiting.
- Symptoms that develop in the dying phase related to renal failure.
  - Fluid overload can lead to water-logging of the lungs and a sense of drowning both for the patient and those observing them.
  - Agitation and confusion may be of increased incidence because of uraemia.
  - Convulsions.
  - Adverse drug effects will also be increased due to ESRD, e.g. myoclonic jerks following morphine administration.

• Symptoms already present and remaining troublesome in the
  terminal phase:
  • itch and dry skin;
  • lethargy;
  • restless legs;
  • cramps.

Incidence of symptoms in patients who discontinue dialysis
These are likely to be similar to those of ESRD and those who follow
the conservative pathway with the addition of end of life symptoms.
However, there are few studies that address this in detail. Cohen *et al.*
in a survey of 79 patients showed that 87% needed analgesia, with
40% experiencing pain in the last 24h, one-third agitation, and a quarter
dyspnoea.[1] With the increasing practice of prescribing in anticipation of
symptoms, it is to be hoped that these symptoms will be alleviated more
quickly and effectively.

Reference
1 Cohen LM, Germain M, Poppel DM, *et al.* (2000). Dialysis discontinuation and palliative care.
Am J Kidney Dis **36**, 140–4.

Symptom management: pain

Pain is commonly experienced by those approaching death. Renal failure itself does not cause pain but the pain of comorbid conditions will continue. It may be added to by pain produced by immobility resulting in joint tenderness and/or pain from pressure areas. Data from one study in the US found that one-third of patients dying following withdrawal of dialysis experienced extremely severe pain at times, while 40% experienced pain in the last 24h. For detailed pain management see Chapter 6.

Management principles

The principles discussed are relevant for all end of life symptoms; those for pain follow the WHO analgesic ladder detailed in Chapter 6, and will include the following.

- Good assessment of the cause(s):
  - including history and examination;
  - diagnosis of cause and type of pain.
- Consideration of psychological and spiritual issues for the patient.
- Use of an approach tailored to the individual.
- A management plan of care with explanation to patient:
  - realistic goal setting.
- The balance of pain relief against adverse effects by:
  - monitoring for efficacy and toxicity;
  - careful titration: adjusting drugs and doses according to response.
- Frequent reassessment of response.
- Use of anticipatory prescribing, which includes ensuring drugs are available to the patient by an appropriate route.

Though timescales may be short and the precise cause of pain may not be clear, it as important to consider causes of pain, such as bowel colic, for which non-opioid treatment is effective. However, as time is of the essence the assessment may need truncating in order to achieve a rapid relief of symptoms with frequent monitoring until pain control is achieved.

Where psychological or spiritual distress impacts on pain control it may be necessary to attempt to resolve these issues before pain control can be achieved. Conversely, there are times when the relief of severe pain is necessary to enable the patient to focus on other issues that are greatly troubling them.

Which opioid and which route?

If the patient can swallow and does not find swallowing medication a burden then the oral route can be used (see Chapter 6). At the end of life when the patient is no longer able to swallow, the subcutaneous route is recommended: it is the least painful and provides a rapid and smooth onset of action. Step 2 analgesia is omitted and step 3 drugs that can be given subcutaneously are used instead, starting at low doses in the opioid-naive. The metabolites of morphine are known to accumulate in renal failure. M6G, a minor metabolite, but clinically the most important due to its potency as an analgesic is likely to be the cause of adverse effects particularly sedation, delirium, and myoclonus.

Agitation and hyperalgesia can also occur in patients being given morphine. The alternative opioids, fentanyl or alfentanil, are recommended when the subcutaneous route is used as this group of drugs have no active metabolites. (See also Chapter 6, p. 104 and guidelines on pp. 242–5.)

Parenteral strong opioids at end of life – fentanyl and alfentanil

All patients should have drugs prescribed and available in anticipation of symptoms as these can develop rapidly and cause considerable distress if not alleviated quickly. For as needed (prn) medication fentanyl is the preferred drug, as it has a longer duration of action, 3–4h, than alfentanil, which may provide pain relief for less than 2h. Doses of 12.5–25mcg of fentanyl are usually used SC up to hourly if needed when the dose is being titrated against pain. If the prn dose is ineffective then it can gradually be increased to the lowest effective dose. If a patient needs more than three prn doses in 24h, it is usually necessary to use a syringe driver to deliver the drug continuously over 24h.

In the opioid-naïve, doses as low as 100–250mcg/24h are usually sufficient. The dose in the syringe driver can be adjusted upwards if further prn analgesia is needed. If fentanyl or alfentanil are unavailable ultra low dose morphine, 1.25mg SC prn, can be used as a temporary measure. It will have a longer duration of action than in those with normal renal function and the patient must be monitored for toxicity, particularly agitation and myoclonus. If these occur, no further morphine should be used. See Guidelines on pp. 242–5.

Adjuvant agents

It may be important to continue these while the patient is able to in order to maintain pain relief.

Paracetamol up to 1g qds can be continued, using the rectal route when the patient can no longer swallow, if it is acceptable to them and considered important for ongoing pain control, particularly that from joints or pressure areas.

NSAIDs may also be helpful for joint stiffness, if used carefully. ESRD patients appear to have a greater risk of GI bleeding with NSAIDs, and any residual renal function will decline further. When comfort is paramount and the patient close to death, then it may be appropriate to use NSAIDs judiciously if they are likely to be the most effective agent for pain relief.

Neuropathic agents may need to be continued until death as the common causes of neuropathic pain such as ischaemia and diabetic neuropathy will continue to give symptoms.
- Clonazepam may be useful as an alternative drug if the person is no longer able to swallow their previous neuropathic agent:
  - it can be given SC as either a nocte dose or in a syringe driver;
  - it has a long duration of action, allowing once daily nocte dose;
  - doses of between 500mcg and 1mg per 24h are usually sufficient, but with titration this can be increased to a maximum of 2mg/24h.

- Gabapentin may be continued until the patient can no longer swallow, at end of life:
  - following cessation of dialysis the dose given after the last dialysis will probably last several days and, if further doses are needed, a maximum of 300mg on alternate days is recommended.

Other neuropathic agents should be continued until the person is unable to swallow and clonazepam made available to them if pain returns. If previous neuropathic pain had been very severe, then it may be wise to start clonazepam as soon as they can no longer take their original agent.

Particular painful situations at end of life

Acute rejection of transplanted kidney

The patient who is dying from rejection of a transplanted kidney, and who has decided not to return to dialysis may develop severe pain in the kidney with associated 'toxicity' from cytokine release. Anti-rejection therapy may be continued as long as feasible, but may need to be replaced with steroids such as dexamethasone, which can be given subcutaneously. Analgesia may also be needed to treat the pain.

Pericarditis with or without effusion

Chest pain with an audible rub may indicate this complication of uraemia. The pain should be managed in the usual way but steroids such as prednisolone 20mg daily may contribute to a reduction in inflammation and therefore pain—again this could be converted to SC dexamethasone if needed.

- 20mg prednisolone is equivalent to 3mg dexamethasone.

Painful procedures

Washing patients may be painful at the end of life as well as carrying out any dressings that may be necessary. Such activities can, where possible, be anticipated and SC fentanyl (or alfentanil, which can also be given buccally, if pain relief only required for a very short time) given prior to the activity. See also Chapter 6, pp. 108–9.

Management: dyspnoea and retained secretions

Dyspnoea The causes of dyspnoea include the following.

Fluid overload, including secondary pleural effusions

This is fortunately less common than might be expected in renal failure. However, it can occur and will need active management.

It is unlikely that it would be appropriate to use high dose diuretics at this stage, though consideration would be given to them in the light of the clinical situation and the ease and appropriateness of IV access if the patient is not dying imminently. In the imminently dying the clinical aim is to reduce the distress of the symptom by non-invasive medical means. These can consist of:

- positioning the patient in as upright a position as they can tolerate;
- oxygen;
- cool fan on the face;
- opioids. These work by reducing the sensation of breathlessness and are used as for pain. The recommended parenteral opioid is fentanyl used at 50–100% dose used for pain and given SC as needed up to hourly (or continuously though a syringe driver if it is clear repeated doses will be required);
- benzodiazepines. If dyspnoea is associated with distress and agitation then low dose midazolam, 2.5–5mg SC available hourly can give helpful relief. Again this can be added to a syringe driver. Usually quite low doses such as 5–10mg over 24h are all that are needed.

Pneumonia

In the final days of life any treatment is designed for comfort and relief of symptoms. The patient who is dying and asymptomatic from pneumonia is not going to benefit from antibiotics. For someone dying, but symptomatic, dyspnoea can be managed as above. In addition, if in pain, analgesia is indicated. The judicious use of rectal paracetamol may help if distressing pyrexia present, but if symptoms are not relieved by the above means consideration of antibiotics should be given.

Acidosis This is a theoretical risk for patients, particularly those who stop dialysis and their normal drugs. However, it is not usually justified to use the invasive approach of IV bicarbonate, etc. but rather to give symptomatic relief for distress and dyspnoea as described above.

Generalized weakness

This may be a cause of dyspnoea, and is likely to contribute to the high percentage of hospice patients who are reported to experience the symptom at end of life, many without other specific physical cause.

General physical measures of support, particularly positioning, will be important here, and the use of medication is not usually necessary.

Retained respiratory secretions

'Death rattle', the noisy rattling breathing that occurs at the end of life for between a quarter to a half of hospice patients, may be more common in renal patients especially those who are anuric. How much, or indeed if, this distresses the patient is unknown, as usually the patient is unconscious at this time. It does distress a proportion of relatives and staff. This in itself would not normally be an indication for medical intervention as side-effects from the drugs used might inadvertently cause distress, e.g. through drying the mouth, or through paradoxical agitation or unwanted sedation if hyoscine hydrobromide used. In the patient with renal failure, however, the early symptoms from secretions in the respiratory tract may presage more symptomatic fluid overload and so it is customary to address them early in the hopes of preventing worse symptoms before death. Either hyoscine butylbromide or glycopyrronium are suitable drugs that may have to be used at maximum doses. Neither crosses the blood–brain barrier and they are therefore less likely to cause paradoxical agitation than hyoscine hydrobromide.

Management: agitation, delirium, and neurological problems

Agitation, delirium

Delirium is very common at end of life, occurring in up to 85% of patients of hospitalized terminally ill patients. This high incidence is likely to be reflected in the ESRD population because of the metabolic disturbances.

Causes include:
- uraemia and metabolic disturbance;
- hypoxia;
- drug toxicity;
- infection;
- alcohol or other drug withdrawal;
- existential distress.

Management
General measures are those for the confused patient:
- keeping stimuli to a minimum;
- familiar surroundings;
- gentle re-orientation;
- minimize changes of staff;
- exclusion of reversible physical causes;
- presence of familiar family or friends and as small a group of professional carers as possible.

Specific measure
- Antipsychotic medication such as low dose haloperidol 0.5–1mg SC prn up to 8-hourly or given initially more frequently until relief obtained.
- Benzodiazepines may be indicated (see guidelines, pp. 242–5). Midazolam 2.5–5mg SC works rapidly and can be repeated as needed. If more prolonged sedation is needed then it can be put in a syringe driver. Low doses are usually sufficient, particularly as there is increased sensitivity.

Neurological problems

Convulsions occur in about 10% patients and it is usually possible to control this with midazolam, though other measures such as IV lorazepam may be necessary.

Myoclonic jerks may vary from the occasional jerk to distressing and quite violent spontaneous jerks causing patients to drop or 'throw' cups of tea. They suggest a lowered seizure threshold. Causes include:
- toxicity from the morphine metabolite, morphine-6-glucuronide;
- gabapentin toxicity with myoclonus;
- antipsychotic agents such as clozepine.

If drug-induced, the drug should be stopped. An alternative opioid such as fentanyl instead of morphine can be used (see above). Clonazepam can be used if gabapentin is the cause—both to treat the myoclonus and as an antineuropathic pain measure. It can be given for immediate symptomatic relief both as SC injections and in a syringe driver if indicated.

Management: nausea and vomiting

It is well known that uraemia can cause nausea and vomiting. However, most patients dying of or with ESRD will be used to living with uraemia and it is likely many will have developed tolerance to this effect. (It is also possible that chronic nausea has been accepted as part of the chronic illness and therefore neither recorded nor managed.) At cessation of dialysis, uraemia will worsen and nausea also may worsen or appear for the first time. An assessment of other likely causes should be made and the symptom managed vigorously. As the commonest basis for the nausea is stimulation of the chemoreceptor trigger zone, appropriate antiemetics include haloperidol (if not otherwise contraindicated) at reduced dose or the broad spectrum antiemetic, levomepromazine, at ultra low dose. 5mg once or twice a day or in a syringe driver is often sufficient without causing excess sedation.

Patients who feel nauseated for other reasons should have antiemesis tailored to the probable cause, e.g. metoclopramide for gastric stasis (see Table 7.2, pp. 130–1), or should continue on previously effective antiemetics. If necessary these can be given SC.

Antiemetics that can be given SC include:
- metoclopramide (maximum 40mg/24h);
- cyclizine (may choose to avoid as it dries the mouth and may crystallize with hyoscine butylbromide and alfentanil);
- haloperidol;
- levomepromazine.

If uncertain of the cause, levomepromazine is a broad spectrum antiemetic with a good track record of efficacy and can be effective at very low doses such as 5mg/24h.

Symptom management: syringe drivers and anticipatory prescribing

Indications for using a syringe driver

Constant symptoms requiring repeated administration of medication are often best managed by means of continuous SC medication at end of life. Precise timing of the introduction of a syringe driver will be determined by discussion with the patient but specific indications include:
• the patient is no longer able to swallow medication;
• the patient is too exhausted to repeatedly swallow medication;
• unpleasant nausea or vomiting.

The doses necessary can be calculated from previous requirement of prn medication; prn medication should continue to be available to them. See also guidelines on pp. 242–5.

Anticipatory prescribing

The key to ensuring good symptom control is the prescription and availability of drugs to relieve symptoms when they occur, wherever the patient is being cared for. This is particularly so if the person is in their own home or a nursing home where it is important that drugs are available at short notice for sudden onset of severe and distressing symptoms. A small supply of drugs to cover the main likely emergencies at end of life, namely, pain, agitation/distress, retained secretions, and nausea or vomiting, can be kept in the home with an up-to-date prescription so a district, hospice, or Marie Curie nurse can administer them as needed without delay.

End of life symptom control guidelines

> The aim of treatment is the comfort of the patient and the support of those close to them

This section gives guidelines for the care of patients with established renal failure who are in the last days of life and a detailed summary of symptom control for these patients.

- Use these guidelines when the whole team, the patient, and the family agree that the patient is in the last days of their life.
- This is a guide to treatment. Practitioners should exercise their own professional judgement according to the clinical situation.
- It is helpful to have considered the following questions.

  - Do the patient, family, and healthcare professionals recognize that the end of life is approaching?
  - Has the preferred place of care been discussed with patient and family and their wishes recorded?
  - Have all unnecessary investigations, including blood tests and routine monitoring, e.g. BP, been discontinued?
  - Have all non-palliative medications been discontinued and is comfort care, particularly care of mouth and skin, in place?
  - *Are the drugs needed for palliation prescribed by route appropriate for the patient's situation and are they available as needed?*
  - Have the patient and family been asked about their cultural, spiritual, and religious needs at this time?

Pain control

> For good symptom control prn medication should be prescribed for likely symptoms *even when the patient is asymptomatic*

All of the drugs listed in this section should be given SC unless otherwise specified.

- All patients should have a strong opioid prescribed to be available as needed (prn).
- Recommendation: fentanyl 12.5–25mcg SC up to hourly.

Patient in pain: opioid-naive

Pain intermittent.
- See box on 'Adjuvant drugs'.
- Prescribe fentanyl 12.5 or 25mcg SC as needed up to hourly.
- After 24h or sooner, review medication.
- If patient still in pain set up SC syringe driver (SD) to run over 24h.
  - Starting SD dose usually fentanyl 100–250mcg/24h.
  - 25mcg of fentanyl SC is approximately equivalent to 2mg SC morphine or 1.5mg SC diamorphine.

Pain continuous
- Start continuous SC infusion in syringe driver with fentanyl.
- Starting dose depends of frailty of patient and severity of pain: 100–250mcg/24h fentanyl.
- Prescribe prn medication, SC fentanyl one-tenth of the 24h dose, which can be given hourly.
- Increase or decrease dose in syringe driver depending on response or side-effects.

Adjuvant drugs for specific indications

- Bowel colic. Consider hyoscine butylbromide (Buscopan®) 20mg SC stat and up to 240mg/24h
- Joint stiffness, bedsores. Consider rectal paracetamol or NSAID
- Neuropathic pain. Consider clonazepam 0.5mg SC prn or nocte; can be given 12-hourly
- Associated anxiety and distress. Add midazolam 2.5mg SC hourly. A combination of midazolam and fentanyl or alfentanil can be very effective in agitated patients who are in pain

Patient in pain: already on strong opioid (See box below if patient already on a fentanyl patch).
- If the patient is on another strong opioid need to convert to dose equivalent of fentanyl—or alfentanil if > 600mcg fentanyl/24h required. See box on 'Supporting information', p. 244, and contact palliative care team.

Opioid-responsive pain
- Increase present dose by 25–30%, *or*
- add up previous day's prn doses and add to the regular dose (do not include doses used for specific movement-related pain, e.g. dressing change or washing),
- *plus prn medication*, SC fentanyl 12.5–25mcg hourly (see above).

Pain poorly responsive to opioid
- Consider adjuvant (see box above or contact local palliative care services).

Patient with a fentanyl patch

- If the pain is controlled *continue* with the patch
- If pain is not controlled, continue with patch, titrating additional analgesia with prn or continuous SC fentanyl or alfentanil

If uncertain, please contact senior medical, nursing, or pharmacy staff on your team or your local palliative care services

Supporting information for pain control and other symptom management

- Fentanyl and alfentanil are suggested as alternative strong opioids to morphine for patients in renal failure as they have no active metabolites with the potential to cause symptomatic and distressing toxicity such as myoclonic jerks and agitation
- In the opioid-naive patient successful pain relief can be achieved with low doses, e.g. fentanyl 100–200mcg/24h without excess sedation
- SC fentanyl is about 75 times as potent as SC morphine so:
  - 200mcg/24h SC fentanyl is *approximately* equivalent to 30mg/24h oral or 15mg/24h SC morphine and 4mg/24h oral hydromorphone
- Alfentanil is 1/4–1/5 as potent as fentanyl, and 10 times as potent as SC diamorphine or 15 times as potent as SC morphine. Use when doses of fentanyl exceed 600mcg/24h as fentanyl less soluble and the volume too great for the syringe driver
- We do not usually recommend alfentanil for dose titration as it has a very short duration of action (30–60min). It is useful for painful procedures, however. Suggested dose for patient on SC alfentanil would be approximately 1/10th the 24-hour dose
- Fentanyl and alfentanil can be mixed with all the common drugs in a syringe driver, though care should be taken with alfentanil and cyclizine as it may crystallize
- Clonazepam can be given SC and may provide a useful adjuvant for neuropathic pain. As there is increased sensitivity to benzodiazepines in ESRD, titrate carefully against toxicity, starting with 500mcg/24h to a maximum of 2mg/24h
- NSAIDs may worsen renal function. However, for patients in the last days of life this may not be relevant and comfort is paramount
- Tramadol preferred to codeine for step 2 analgesia as idiosyncratic occurrence of respiratory depression with codeine for step 2. Maximum 24h tramadol dose of 100mg. Dextropropoxyphene and dihydrocodeine should be avoided
- All strong opioids should be monitored carefully, recognizing that pain and the patient's clinical condition often change rapidly
- If the patient develops Cheyne–Stokes respiration, it is usually a terminal event and the patient is often unconscious. It is important to explain this and reassure the relatives that we do not believe the patient is suffering at this time

If uncertain, please contact senior medical, nursing, or pharmacy staff on your team or your local palliative care services

At this stage the goal is relief of symptoms and the cause of the symptom may not be relevant.

Retained respiratory tract secretions

- Symptoms absent: hyoscine butylbromide 20mg SC stat and 2-hourly prn.
- Symptoms present: hyoscine butylbromide 40–120mg/24h SC via syringe driver (SD) + 20mg 2-hourly prn up to 240mg/24h.

Terminal restlessness and agitation

- Symptom absent: midazolam 2.5mg SC up to hourly prn. NB. Increased cerebral sensitivity in ESRD.
- Symptom present: midazolam 2.5mg SC up to hourly prn. If two or more doses required, consider syringe driver with 10–20mg/24h + prn dose.

Nausea and vomiting

- Symptoms absent.
  - If already taking effective antiemetic, e.g. metoclopramide, cyclizine, haloperidol, or levomepromazine, it can be given in a syringe driver over 24h.
  - If not taking an antiemetic, prescribe levomepromazine 5mg SC prn 8-hourly.
- Symptoms present. Start levomepromazine 5mg SC prn up to 8-hourly or start 5–10mg/24h by continuous SC infusion with further two doses of 5mg/24h SC prn.

Shortness of breath

The following may be helpful whatever the cause.

- Positioning the patient. A cool fan on the face. Oxygen, if hypoxic, and the reassuring presence of family or staff.
- Strong opioids such as fentanyl used at half to the full recommended dose for pain. Use prn up to hourly or in syringe driver if repeated doses needed.
- Benzodiazepines such as midazolam 2.5mg SC can be given up to hourly if shortness of breath associated with anxiety or panic attacks.

Fluid overload

This is less common than might be expected but is very distressing if it occurs. Use guidance for dyspnoea (p. 234 and above) for symptomatic help or consider the following.

- Sublingual nitrates.
- If appropriate, consider high dose furosemide or ultrafiltration to comfort.

Control of symptoms other than pain

For the symptoms described on this page all patients should have prn medication prescribed and available

Dialysis at end of life

Even after recognizing that the patient is nearing the end of life, it may be appropriate to continue dialysis. Various factors do need to be considered, though, for both HD and PD.

Haemodialysis at end of life

- Vascular access may be problematic requiring frequent (and often unpleasant) catheter insertions.
- Patients become more dependent.
  - Need transport to and from HD.
  - May no longer be able to manage at home and will have to consider moving to a nursing home.
  - Increasing problems of hypotension on dialysis with risk of cardiac arrest.
- Increasing dementia or confusion may make patient less able to cope with dialysis procedure.

Peritoneal dialysis at end of life

- Patient often too sick to carry out self-care treatment.
- May no longer be able to live independently.
- Nutrition.
- Increased risk of peritonitis.
  - PD may be being performed by ward nurses.
  - Patient technique may be poor.
- Transfer to HD may have to be considered.

Preferred place of care

The Preferred Place of Care document is a patient-held record, designed to record and monitor patient and carer choices and services received by all terminally ill patients. It aims to give patients and carers choices and to aid communication between visiting professionals. The desired place cannot be guaranteed and the document also acknowledges that patients may change their minds during the course of their final illness and aims to accommodate this. Patients are encouraged once they have completed such a document to take it into hospital with them if they are admitted to help with future care planning. Discussions around preferred place of care should take place with all patients in whom death is expected in days or weeks and these should be documented, and acted on where possible. Support must be given particularly to patients who are not able to achieve their preferred setting for their final illness and who may experience great distress because of this.

The nursing perspective of end of life care in the renal setting

Overview

- *Patients dying in the renal unit have often been known to staff for many years*
- *Staff have built up long term professional relationships with such patients through their illness at clinic attendances, inpatient stays and through dialysis sessions often conducted over many years*
- *When such well known patients enter the end of life phase of care the familiarity between staff and patient built up over such a long time poses both opportunities and also challenges for staff working in renal units*
  - *Opportunities: Patients entering the end of life phase are able to do so in the knowledge that they will be looked after by staff well known to them which can be a source of great comfort*
  - *Challenges: For staff the change in goals of care from active intervention to comfort, and the emotional impact of loosing patients and their families who have become friends over the years can be emotionally demanding*

Practicalities

On most UK renal units at admission every patient is allocated to a trained nurse who has overall responsibility for ongoing care. This responsibility will be handed over to another nurse at the end of each shift. The allocated nurse will liaise with the patient, family and the multidisciplinary team and be central to the provision of care for each patient. She will act as the patient's advocate in multi-professional discussions and will often have the major contact with family members.

When it becomes clear that a patient's condition is deteriorating, the patient, family and professional team will have discussions, usually over several days concerning the choices for ongoing care. The process of conducting such discussions in a sensitive and open manner is crucial to ensure that the greatest chance possible is given to arriving at consensus decisions involving, patient, family and staff. If it is considered appropriate to stop dialysis, many units, following discussion with patient and family, will commence the patient on an integrated care pathway in an attempt to ensure that end of life care is optimal.

Care pathways

Contribution of an the integrated care pathway to end of life care of patients in a renal unit;

- Facilitates regular nursing assessment of patient comfort
- Aids recording of symptoms
- Enhances nurse confidence in their ability to treat symptoms promptly
- Reduces volume of paperwork to be filled out
- Encourages nurses to focus attention on caring for the emotional and spiritual needs of the family as well as the patient

Stopping dialysis

During the first few days following cessation of dialysis many renal patients will still be able to eat small amounts and take oral fluids. This is encouraged until the patient no longer wishes to eat or drink. If a patient was receiving dialysis through a temporary line this usually should be removed to be less burdensome for the patient whereas a long term dialysis patient's permanent fistula or graft causes no discomfort when not being used and would need no further intervention.

Many renal patients choose to stay in the unit where they already know the staff. Others may be discharged to nursing homes or hospices if such placement can be arranged. If the patient and family would like end of life care to be at home meticulous communication between the hospital renal and palliative care teams and the community primary and palliative care services using the most effective means possible is essential in order to plan and set up a package of home terminal care at very short notice.

Death on the renal unit

When death occurs on the ward, after verification; nursing staff complete last offices and the body is taken to the mortuary. The patient's GP is informed of the death. It may also be important to inform sensitively other patients on the unit of what has happened, particularly if the patient who has did has been well known by other patients.

Changing focus of care

The biggest challenge for nursing staff is managing the change from active treatments, like dialysis, to comfort care with support of the relatives as well as the patient.

The length of time supporting patients and families in the renal context through the dying phase is variable, but tends to be longer than is common in other conditions, sometimes up to 14 days or more. The family needs sensitive ongoing support and other specialists including those from palliative care, psychology and the chaplaincy team can help with this.

At the time of death it is important that patients and families are afforded privacy and dignity, and awareness of support. When informing the family that the patient has died it is important that clear and unambiguous language is used and euphemisms avoided. It is also important that the professional informing the family of the death does not leave the room immediately but stays to offer support to the family.

Families can also be helped in other ways, including;

* Advice and instruction on what they need to do next (including written leaflets)
* Nursing staff can accompany the family to view the body in the chapel of rest
* Contact with the hospital's chaplaincy or pastoral support team can be made if not previously in touch

Team support

In recognition of the stress that can occur for nurses and other team members there are a number of ways staff can be supported
- The opportunities of informal support where staff can talk through difficulties with each other in the normal contact periods of each day
- Regular team supervision/debrief sessions with the psychologist where staff have the opportunity, in a safe and controlled environment, to talk about the stresses of the ward
- Attendance by a member of the hospital team at the funeral of long standing patients
- Follow up of family members with a phone call a few days later. See also chap 14
- A formal post death audit on all deaths on the unit can be a very useful forum for looking at the quality of end of life care, and acknowledging areas of care which can be improved or which need to be encouraged. The value of such meetings is maximized if they are viewed as a priority by all key staff working on the unit, attendance expected, minutes taken, and outcomes reviewed and monitored

Summary: main principles of end of life care

Death is either expected or likely for a significant number of patients with ESRD.

- Their care at this stage of their illness is an integral part of the work of a renal team; its importance cannot be overestimated as it is crucial for the alleviation of suffering where possible and it is the basis for bereavement support for the family and friends of those who die.
- Fundamental to end of life care are careful communication, meticulous attention to symptom control, and regard to the psychological, social, and spiritual needs of the patient, family, and carers.
- Anticipation of symptoms with the appropriate prescription and provision of medication and advance planning of future care will all contribute to this.

For summary of practical aspects see pp. 242–5.

Further reading

Chambers EJ (2004). End of life care, the terminal phase. In *Supportive care for the renal patient*, (ed. EJ Chambers, M Germain, E Brown), pp. 255–65. Oxford University Press, Oxford.

Integrated care pathway for end of life care

The integrated care pathway for end of life care, developed by Ellershaw and team from Liverpool,[1] aims to build on best practice in end of life care as developed by the hospice movement by providing a framework of care so that this standard is translatable into all settings. It hopes to empower doctors and nurses as they care for people at the end of life, by setting goals of care and to facilitate multiprofessional communication, documentation, and audit.

There are clear steps for organizations who wish to introduce the pathway and a pathway specific to patients with end-stage renal failure is currently being piloted across the UK.

It is hoped that by measurable improvement in the documentation of end of life care there will come actual improvement in the care both of the patient and their relatives but also greater confidence and job satisfaction for the professional carers as the importance of the care of those who are dying is recognized.

The goals of the renal pathway remain the same as those for the generic one. Differences include the following.

- Units may start using the pathway at cessation of dialysis, i.e. earlier than the last 72h of life, because:
  - once a patient has stopped dialysis death is certain;
  - principles of care can be applied as soon as needed;
  - enables team to discuss preferred place of care when patient more likely to be well enough to indicate preferences;
  - documentation of patient preferences and whether achieved can be used to guide resource planning.
- Symptom control guidelines are modified:
  - to account for different drug usage in renal failure;
  - to include symptoms more common in renal failure.

The care pathway is divided into three sections:
- initial assessment and care of the dying patient;
- ongoing care of dying patient;
- care of the family and carers after death.

Initial assessment

The initial assessment includes agreement between renal team, patient, and family that the patient is at the end of their life.

The criteria for diagnosing dying, and hence commencing the pathway in the generic document, i.e. that the patient is bedbound or semicomatose or only able to take sips of water, or unable to take tablets, are not necessarily applicable to the renal patient stopping dialysis. In this specific situation the pathway is often started once the decision to stop dialysis is made. However, other key aspects of the pathway apply, including:
- assessment of symptoms;
- review of medication;

- the prescribing of anticipatory drugs for potential symptoms;
- cessation of routine blood tests and investigations;
- institution of comfort care.

Importantly, the care pathway also addresses the insight of patient and family as to the situation, their spiritual and psychological needs, and the physical needs of the carers, who may be spending considerable time in hospital and need access to facilities such as bathroom and overnight accommodation for themselves.

An adapted initial assessment sheet is seen in Fig. 12.1

Ongoing care of dying patient is documented in a single set of multidisciplinary notes, with a minimum of 4-hourly checks on symptoms, and twice daily checks on psychological and spiritual aspects of care, including the needs of the carers.

Care of the family and carers after death This section is important as it ensures the ongoing care of the bereaved in terms of practical information about what needs to be done and information about bereavement resources.

Reference

1 Ellershaw JE, Wilkinson S (eds.) (2003). *Care of the dying: a pathway to excellence.* Oxford University Press, Oxford.

IF PATIENT HAS RECENTLY STOPPED DIALYSIS COMPLETE THE FOLLOWING

Was there a clear reason?   Yes ☐   No ☐

IF yes please state the reason:

Not tolerating dialysis   ☐
Deterioration in spite of dialysis   ☐
Patient's wishes   ☐
Patient unconscious   ☐
Other . . . .

Has reason for stopping dialysis been discussed with the patient?
          Yes ☐   No ☐   N/A ☐
Has stopping dialysis been discussed with the next of kin?
          Yes ☐   No ☐   N/A ☐
Have the patient and family been asked about preferred place of care?
          Yes ☐   No ☐   N/A ☐
What is the preferred place of care?
          Hospital ☐   Hospice ☐
          Home ☐   Continuing care nursing home ☐
Was the preferred place of care achieved?
          Yes ☐   No ☐   N/A ☐

Fig 12.1 Possible additional information to be added to renal integrated care pathway.

Spiritual and religious care

Introduction

The care of any patient and specifically of one who is approaching death must encompass the physical, psychological, social, and spiritual aspects of that person.

Spirituality is about making sense of what is happening to someone. It has to do with an individual's sense of peace and connection to others and their belief about the meaning of life. It is likely to be heightened at times of crisis such as facing a life-limiting illness or in the face of certain death.

Spirituality may be found through an organized religion or in other ways.

Religion is defined as a specific set of beliefs and practices, usually within an organized group. It may contain ritual of worship or expression of faith, which varies with different beliefs and which helps that individual express their spirituality. It is important to differentiate the two, as a person who has no religious belief or needs may welcome spiritual care that affirms their humanity and supports their exploration of meaning, while not wishing any religious ritual.

It is helpful to know if the patient has any spiritual or religious beliefs or practices, and how much of a source of strength they are to that individual and therefore how they might help him or her during their remaining life. It is not uncommon for transient loss of faith at this time and patients should be asked if they wish to see a chaplain or religious leader.

End of life issues can challenge a patient's beliefs or religious values resulting in high levels of spiritual distress. Some believe their illness is a punishment for some previous misdemeanour, which may result in increased distress and loss of faith.

Spiritual care

> Spiritual care is not just the facilitation of an appropriate ritual but engaging with an individual's search for existential meaning, as reflected in the existential domain of the McGill quality of life questionnaire[1]
>
> P Speck

Spiritual care is embedded within the holistic care of patient, family, and professional staff that palliative care embraces, yet it is often omitted or only has lip service paid to it. This may be through ignorance, embarrassment, lack of confidence, or fear of opening a conversation that the individual either has not the time or the personal resources to deal with. This is worrying and unnecessary as all members of the multidisciplinary renal team who care for the dying patient can reach out to their patients' spiritual needs through normal practice and contact with patients. Often patients' spiritual needs are expressed at a time when pastoral or chaplaincy staffs are not present. Frequently, this will be when people are at their most vulnerable, such as while being washed or having dressings changed, yet individuals will trust the staff member sufficiently to express their deep concerns—maybe with a question relating to their death.

Such opportunities are precious and should be responded to. This may involve holding on to the silence, or listening and enabling the patient to continue their questioning or tell their story, or through touch and an honest meeting of the eyes. For the patient it is the professional 'staying with them' at a time of need or distress that counts. It is also possible to offer further spiritual support from chaplaincy staff if the patient wishes, but it is equally important not to miss the opportunity in everyday practice.

Spirituality and spiritual distress

- Spirituality relates to the way people make sense of the world around them.
- It is about finding meaning in life.
- The knowledge or fear of the closeness of death is likely to bring those aspects of our being sharply into focus.
- Everyone has a spiritual dimension, though not all have spiritual needs.
- If spiritual distress is not recognized and attended to, it may lead to difficult symptom control, particularly pain control.
- Spiritual distress may express itself as terminal agitation or difficult and unrelieved pain.
- Relief of spiritual distress may be crucial to the 'healing' of an individual as they approach their death, and such healing will enhance their quality of life and aid symptom control.

Religious care

Religious care enables the person to express their spirituality through appropriate ritual and religious practice. A recently published audit of care of renal patients at the end of life demonstrated the wide variety of religious beliefs or none held by the patients in that unit; nearly 1/3 were Christian but 44% were of unknown religion with the remainder of the patients distributed between five other faith communities.[2] These proportions will vary according to the geographical site of the unit. This audit suggested clinical staff failed at times to take these needs into account and demonstrates the need for understanding of religious customs and practices. For all people, however, personal events and beliefs through their lives may shape the approach to the end of life. Loss of faith, actions in the past for which they feel unforgiven, and actions by others, whom they have not been able to forgive may lead to spiritual distress, which can be helped with either spiritual help such as listening without judgement to someone's story, or religious help using rituals and customs appropriate to their faith.

Reference

1 Speck P, Higginson IJ, Addington-Hall JM (2004). Spiritual needs in health care. *Br Med J* **329**, 123–4.
2 Noble H, Rees K (2006) Caring for people who are dying on renal wards: a retrospective study. EDTNA/ERCA Journal 89–92.

Assessing spiritual and religious needs

- Assessment of spiritual needs should take place prior to the dying phase as patients are unlikely to have the energy to address such issues and maintain concentration as death draws closer.
- Open questions such as 'how do you deal or cope with life when faced with tough and difficult situations?' or 'is there anything that gives you a particular sense of meaning to your life?' let the patient know you are willing to engage in a discussion about spiritual matters and can be used to open a discussion.
- It is also important to gauge how important this is in the person's life, so you might ask 'how important is this (or your faith) in your life?'.
- If the person tells you of their faith this gives you the opportunity to ask if they would like to see a 'faith leader' and if so to ensure the chaplaincy team is aware of this.
- They should also be asked how they would like these matters to be dealt with in their health care or could be asked 'are there any particular religious customs I need to know about to help you?'.

Giving spiritual support includes:
- being led by the patient;
- listening actively;
- using silence;
- avoiding judgement;
- liaison with appropriate pastoral support or religious leaders.

Spiritual and religious well-being is associated with quality of life with some research showing that these beliefs can promote a more positive mental attitude that can enhance patients remaining quality of life by:
- reducing anxiety;
- reducing depression;
- reducing a sense of isolation and 'aloneness';
- facilitating better acceptance and adjustment to their illness.

Spiritual distress may contribute to the patient's inability to cope with end of life issues. Knowing the role that religion and spirituality plays in the patient's life may help caregivers understand the beliefs that affect the patient's responses to end of life issues.

Assessing spiritual and religious needs: a practical summary

- Try to ensure privacy and sufficient time
- Ask what is important in the person's life or if anything gives their life meaning
- Find out how important this is to them
- If a patient tells you of their faith, ask what kind of support they would like
- Discover what if any religious practices are important for their spiritual well being, e.g. opportunity to pray in a particular way
- Find out if there are particular things to be avoided or others that are important in their faith life
- Find out if they have a minister of religion whom they would like contacted at any time
- At an appropriate time ascertain whether they have an up to date will and, if not, if they wish to produce one
- Be prepared to discuss their funeral wishes if they wish
- When the time is right enquire about practice around death itself and afterwards—this will depend on the person's response to previous questions

Cultural issues and spiritual support

In every culture loss is accompanied by grief, although it may be expressed in a variety of ways

In a multicultural society patients have different attitudes towards discussing death. No individual can be separated from the context in which they live, be it family, medical, or wider social contexts. It can be a frightening and bewildering experience for those who do not speak the same language as those who care for them, and patients can be left feeling very isolated and misunderstood.

The cultural and religious backgrounds of patients may play an integral role in their interpretation of death and the coping mechanisms they use. Many view death as a transition rather than extinction so it can be seen that religion and spirituality can influence one's concept of death and dying by offering a reason for being and a framework in which to interpret the inevitable.

Communication

Effective communication is needed when working in a cross-cultural setting. Otherwise one cannot check that a patient has fully understood the implications of end of life care discussions.

We need to recognize the following.

- Mourning behaviour and rituals must be understood within the bereaved individual's religious and cultural background.
- Having prior knowledge of cultural issues, including how the patient's cultural, spiritual, or religious beliefs influence the way they think about caring for the dying, avoids burdening the patient or the family with the additional role of being educators.
- We may not know how patients maintain good health, what they believe to be the cause of their illness, and whether religion or spiritual beliefs play a role in their illness, but we can establish this by admitting we are unfamiliar with their culture and asking how best we can help them.
- If language barriers are hampering good communication, the services of an independent interpreter should be sought.

All people expect their cultural values and way of life to be respected and understood, which is why we should try to think in terms of similarities between cultures rather than differences.

Religious practices of different faiths in relation to end of life care

See Table 13.1 for a summary of end of life practices of different faiths.

It is not possible to cover all shades of each religion in this short section, it is important *always to ask* the individual and family what their personal practice and religious needs are, and not to assume that they will conform to a 'norm' as described here or in other texts

Buddhism There are a number of different schools of Buddhism, any of which may be represented among renal patients and all of whom practise meditation. Buddhism teaches the inevitability of death. Therefore, a practitioner is likely to be calm and dignified as they face death. Though relief of pain is acceptable, analgesics and sedatives may be declined towards the end of life, and sometimes earlier, so as to die with a clear mind.

Euthanasia is rejected but withdrawal of medical intervention when death is near is not seen as immoral so discontinuing dialysis for the indications discussed in Chapter 12 would be permitted.

Customs at end of life include:
- inviting a Buddhist teacher or monk to be present with the patient;
- peace and quiet for meditation to ensure a calm state of mind as dying:
  - single sex room particularly for monks;
- listening to Buddhist chants as death approaches.

Christianity Within Christianity there are also a number of denominations with different traditions. Central to Christianity is the belief that Jesus Christ was the son of God and that he rose from the dead following crucifixion and thereby atoned for the sins of humanity. Christians believe in life after death. Attitudes to death will vary from a rejoicing acceptance to great distress, and all shades between; distress may be associated with feelings of guilt concerning sins unforgiven or a loss of faith. Many (but not all) are helped by seeing a priest or minister of their own or similar denomination for prayer, which may be accompanied by confession, absolution, holy communion, or anointing. It is important that a Roman Catholic receives the sacrament of the sick from a Roman Catholic priest.

Analgesia and sedation can be accepted for relief of pain and suffering. However, some Christians may wish to remain clear in their thinking and decline medication, or delay its use to give time for repentance or reconciliation. Intentionally bringing about death is forbidden; however, attempts to prolong life at all costs are not commensurate with Christian beliefs either.

Customs at end of life include:
- the sacrament of confession with absolution;
- receiving communion;

- laying on of hands;
- anointing with oil;
- prayer with patient and family.

Hinduism Hinduism is a family of beliefs embracing diversity of traditions but with common beliefs relating to transition to another life either with reincarnation, life in heaven with God, or absorption into Brahman. A good death is an important part of spiritual life. Religious life plays a significant part in physical life and in this context suffering can be seen as a reflection of wrongs committed.

Purification of the body is very important, particularly to bathe in running water, as part of a daily routine. Many will wish to do so before praying in the morning. Most Hindus will wish to have physical care carried out by carers of the same sex as themselves and it is important that this is respected.

A good death occurs peacefully in old age, having put affairs in order, said goodbye, and resolved conflict. The 'old age' aspect of a good death can cause problems for younger Hindus who are dying.

Some Hindus will stop eating and drinking as they approach death as purification of body and spirit. Analgesia and sedation may also be declined to keep the mind clear as they prepare for death. Euthanasia is not permitted.

Customs at end of life include:

- placing the mattress on the floor at end of life;
- preference for death at home;
- having family present while dying;
- reading from Hindu holy books and hymns;
- being given Ganges water and Tulsi leaf in the mouth at the time of death;
- family likely to wish to want to wash the body after death.

Islam Followers of Islam, known as Muslims, believe in one God and the presence of prophets to guide the faithful, the last and most influential of whom was Muhammad. They see the historic record of his actions and teachings as tools for interpreting the Qur'an. Muslims also believe in a final day of judgement. 'Islam' means submitting to the will of God. Most Muslims are strict about abiding by Islamic law with respect to diet, prayer, fasting, etc. Modesty is important in nursing care, with a preference for same sex carers. Prayer is said five times a day, facing Mecca and after washing with running water. These aspects of religious life will be important at the end of life and professional carers must ask the patient what their wishes are.

Fasting during Ramadan from dawn to dusk is incumbent on Muslims in health. Many who are terminally ill may choose to fast a certain amount, particularly as it is also a time for resolving disputes. Meals will need to be provided before dawn and after dusk. As fasting includes taking anything into the body, medication may also be declined during the hours of daylight.

Muslims believe in life after death, that suffering is part of God's plan, and accept death as His will. For the individual, as in other religions, this can be a great comfort but also for some a source of guilt and distress.

Table 13.1 End of life customs of the different religions*

Religion	Diet	Particular requirements	Customs around dying	Actions after death	Method of disposal	Autopsy
Buddhism	Many vegetarian	Peace & quiet to allow meditation	Wish to be calm & fully conscious; may request monk to chant	Contact priest immediately; body should not be removed till he arrives	Burial or cremation	May be permitted if religious teacher allows
Christianity	Individual; no forbidden foods	None	May wish to receive absolution, holy communion, or anointing from priest or minister	No special requirements	Burial or cremation	Permitted; with respect to body
Hindu	Strict handling rules; no beef	May prefer mattress on floor; home death preferred	May call Hindu priest for holy rites; Ganges water and Tulsi leaf placed in mouth	Family to wash (if done by health care workers, with permission, must wear gloves); jewellery left with body	Cremation as soon as possible	Is permitted
Islam	Special preparation; vegetarian or 'halal' meat; no pork	Modesty & cleanliness very important. Washing in running water before prayer. Fully dressed at night	If possible to sit or lie facing Mecca; privacy for continued daily prayer; declaration of faith made	Body washed by same sex Muslim; non-Muslims need permission to touch body; body kept covered in clean white cotton garments	Burial only; within 24h	Permitted if required by law

Judaism	Orthodox kosher meals; check individual requirements	Dying person should not be left alone	Those present may recite psalms; rabbi not essential but may be called	Cover body with white sheet; body laid on floor, feet to the door; candle by head	Burial usually as soon as possible	Only if required by law. Minimally invasive; return of organs to body
Sikhism	Usually decline beef & pork; many vegetarian	May like to recite or listen to hymns from Sikh holy book	Should die with God's name being recited	Do not trim hair or beard; cover body with plain white cloth; leave 5 Ks† with body; family members to wash body	Cremation as soon as possible	Permitted if required by law

* The six faith communities described all prohibit euthanasia but allow the withdrawal of futile treatment. Pain relief is also allowed by all, though practitioners may choose to decline it or sedation so as to maintain as clear a mind as possible, and there may be different interpretations of what is allowed by different practitioners.
† Five Ks: kesh. long hair: kachhera. shorts: kanna. small wooden comb: kara. bracelet: kirpan. sword.

Euthanasia is prohibited, but pain relief can be given and futile treatment withdrawn.

Customs at end of life include:
- wish to die facing Mecca (south-east in UK);
- family or other Muslims to recite prayers;
- after death the body only to be touched by Muslims;
- if staff have to touch the body it should be while wearing disposable gloves;
- the person's face should be placed towards the right shoulder.

Judaism The attitude of Jews to death and dying is based on convictions. They believe the body belongs to God and that therefore there is an obligation to try to heal it. Most Jews will want to know the truth about their illness so they can plan well. Jewish law is binding and Jews may wish to consult family or rabbi before making serious treatment decisions.

Suicide and therefore euthanasia are against Jewish law. It is, however, generally permissible to withdraw life-sustaining treatment in the presence of a terminal illness, if in the patient's best interest. Pain control is permissible as long as not given with the intent of shortening life, though patient may prefer to maintain clarity of thought and decline analgesia.

Customs at end of life include the following.
- Attention to the bereaved may be greater than that to dying person.
- A request to see a rabbi is an individual decision and not necessary for ritual.
- Prayers may be said.
- Traditionally, closing the eyes, laying the arms straight, and binding up the lower jaw are done by a family member.
- After death the body is placed on the floor, feet towards the door, covered with a white sheet, and a candle lit.
- The body cannot be moved on the Sabbath (Saturday) so it is important to have anticipated this.
- 'Watchers' stay with the body till burial.

Summary This has been a brief sketch of some of the features of some faiths. Reference to more extensive texts and to the relevant faith community leaders may be necessary to ensure optimal religious care. All hospitals and hospices have access to chaplaincy or pastoral support teams; these will be an important source of information to local teams and should be used.
- The care of the individual is unique and assumptions based on religious faith should not be made.
- Patients and families should be asked their needs and preferences.
- Care teams should endeavour to honour those wishes.

Cultural resources and further reading

Handbook on cultural, spiritual and religious beliefs. www.sdhl.nhs.uk/documents.cultural.html

Lancet Viewpoint Series: End of Life Issues for different religions (2005). Vol. **366**, pp. 682–6, 774–9, 862–5, 952–5, 1045–8, 1132–5, 1235–7.

Speck P, Higginson IJ, Addington-Hall JM (2004). Spiritual needs in health care. *Br Med J* **329**, 123–4.

Caring for the carers

Introduction

> Counsellor: 'How's Ray?'
>
> Wife: 'He's fine—why wouldn't he be with me running around after him day in and day out? Do you know what would be really nice—if once in a while someone actually asked how I was'

The focus of care is naturally first and foremost on the patient and so it is easy to overlook the fact that the losses he or she is experiencing are also being experienced first hand by the patient's close family.

- It is important to recognize the contribution to patient care that family members give—the level of which isn't always fully appreciated by members of the renal team or indeed by the patient. One wife commented, 'If I tell him I have a headache, he says "think yourself lucky that's all you've got to put up with." He would never think to ask me later in the day if it had gone.'
- Families and carers need to be reminded that we do value the working relationship we have with them and we need to address sensitively their reluctance to ask for help and to understand the difficulty they have in accepting it when offered.
- Finally, carers need permission to care for themselves too.

Caregivers are mostly:
- spouses and partners who had no idea when they committed themselves to the relationship that they would be sharing the limitations of a life of chronic illness;
- adult children and grandchildren, particularly when the parent is widowed and living alone with no other support;
- parents when the adult child is still living at home or locally;
- young carers, often the children of single parents.

What is expected from care givers?
- An up to date basic knowledge of renal disease, its treatments, and medical jargon in order to provide the best level of care.
- Monitoring of renal diet and fluid restrictions.
- Ensuring drug regime is adhered to.
- Assisting with personal care and daily living tasks.
- Providing a taxi service to and from the renal unit.
- Liaising with the unit if the patient is unwell or if there are other concerns such as problems with hospital transport.
- Learning new skills both medically and socially.
- Adapting to relationship and role changes.
- No expectation of financial reward for the care given.

In order to identify potential problem areas, we need to make a comprehensive assessment of the carer's social situation to ensure that the planned provision of care is compatible with the home situation and level of support available. This is particularly relevant as we are now treating an increasingly aged population, some of whom may be living with equally

elderly and frail partners or may, of course, be living alone. In such cases the duty of care often falls to close family members because the patient:
- may be unwilling to have 'a stranger' looking after him (i.e. a carer from social services);
- would rather go without than pay for provision of care;
- may think it is their children's responsibility to care for them, or the children themselves may freely volunteer their services without consultation with their own families who may then feel neglected and resentful at the amount of time being spent with the patient.

This often onerous burden and isolation increases the sense of responsibility carers feel in relation to caring for their loved one. Their expressed concerns relate to:
- risk of infection;
- access or any problem that could result in readmission to the unit;
- being criticized that they 'haven't done things right';
- being perceived by unit staff as a 'nuisance';
- not being able to cope with tiredness and fatigue as a result of being constantly vigilant and 'on duty';
- a fear of becoming ill and unable to continue to care;
- not managing feelings of anxiety and foreboding;
- guilt at feeling angry, resentful, and frustrated;
- feeling taken for granted;
- isolation, together with lack of recognition and support;
- acknowledging that sometimes carers want to run away—not from their loved one but from the situation.

Support for carers

Statutory services

There is a lot that can be done do to support carers at this time. Under the Care in the Community Act, both patients and their carers are entitled to an 'assessment of need', which could result in help being offered such as provision of personal care and equipment that would make life easier for the carer. Ideally, the carer assessment should not be carried out in the presence of the patient as this might inhibit an open and honest appraisal of how things are. Information can also be obtained on local carer support groups, respite care, sitting services, and benefit advice.

Patients sometimes 'bully' their families into taking them home before a comprehensive assessment of need has been carried out. It is important to ensure that all loose ends have been tied up prior to discharge home to make sure the carer is not being set up to fail.

The renal team

Renal team members can offer ongoing support to carers by:
- keeping in regular telephone contact;
- face to face meetings at clinic;
- community visits in order see if needs have changed and more support is required;
- 'normalizing' any negative feelings such as anger, frustration, resentment, or fear;
- offering counselling or psychological support, through the renal team and external resources such as the Expert Patient Programme for Carers—'Caring for Me';
- advising what is available locally for practical and emotional support such as:
  - onward referral for hospice or community palliative care; where there is holistic care for patient and carer;
- encouraging carers to share honestly what they can realistically offer their loved one;
- facilitating respite care if available and appropriate;
- being tolerant and understanding of frequent phone calls—recognizing that the carer is clearly struggling and in need of support;
- recognizing that trying to meet the patient's wish to die at home puts enormous strain on carers who need to be reassured that they won't have failed if they are unable to comply or sustain their loved one's wish.

Carer background issues

- Carers mostly do a wonderful job, rarely complain, and seldom ask for help
- The patient and his/her treatment is the main focus of the renal team
- The losses and limitation associated with CKD and the demands of dialysis are experienced by patients and carers alike
- Those without family support have three times the mortality risk of those with highly supportive families
- Carers are often taken for granted—not just by the patient but by renal unit staff too
- They take on this role out of a sense of love and duty having no real appreciation of the commitment involved, or their eligibility for welfare benefits that exist in recognition of their role
- They feel they can't be ill—they can't give in because who would then care for their loved one?

Useful contacts

- Princess Royal Trust (Tel 020 7480 7788) provides free and confidential help for all carers.
- Benefits Enquiry Line (free phone 0800 882200) for advice on attendance allowance, disability living allowance, invalid care allowance, and benefit eligibility in general.
- NKF Helpline (Tel 0845 6010209), who can deal with specific and general enquiries.
- Local patient associations.
- Expert Patient Programme—'Looking After Me'.

Useful websites

www.caresonline.org.uk
www.crossroads.org
www.carers.gov.uk
www.pensionsguide.gov.uk
www.dss.gov.uk

Caring for the professional

'Meanwhile, it seems, the world is suffering from compassion fatigue.'

Salman Rushdie

Long, deep, and meaningful relationships are built with patients and families, who later choose to stop active treatment and embark on end of life care. This change in care aim may impact on the staff who have built up such a relationship. Working in this field can be both rewarding and demanding and staff need to protect themselves against emotional burnout and compassion fatigue.

The long association staff have with renal patients has the potential to render them too central in the lives of both patient and family. This can result in some relatives finding difficulty in 'letting go' even after death. This after-care attachment can manifest in visits to where their loved one was cared for and, whilst offering comfort and solace to the family, it can create a range of mixed emotions with staff members as they try to reconcile the needs of the bereaved family with the needs of a new cohort of patients. And so often the staff's own needs remain completely neglected.

We have to care for patients who are going to die, absorbing their physical and emotional pain on a daily basis. The professional cannot change the fact that the patient has not only to cope with their prognosis but also with subsequent changes in family life, employment, and social contacts. If a patient is still in the angry stage of their grief process, this can be displaced on to staff who find themselves facing hostile outbursts, mood swings, and demanding behaviour—all of which is very hard to handle as it is often taken personally as a criticism of care given.

How do we cope with dissonant emotions that we fear may damage our relationship with a patient at a time when they need compassion and unconditional care? Sometimes there is a tendency to overcompensate, to be overly friendly and devoted, rather than to actually show the patient how we are feeling because it doesn't 'fit' with our professional persona.

This internal conflict, which many staff experience, can result in exhaustion and physical symptoms such as gastrointestinal disturbances, fatigue, insomnia, and headaches. Psychological reactions include depressed mood, irritability, anxiety, rigidity, negativism, and lack of motivation. On a social level it becomes easier to avoid contact with patients or to react impatiently to their constant demands.

Working in a renal unit can be very stressful for the staff primarily because of the psychological burden of continually working with incurably ill patients. Denial is a mechanism often used by staff to avoid burn-out. Patients' behaviour and ways of coping can depend on the way staff deal with their own emotions and it is helpful to develop strategies to prevent burn-out.

Ways to support staff and reduce levels of stress

- Regular staff meetings that address not just the physical symptoms of the patient but also the psychological impact of caring for them.
- Opportunities to debrief and share their experiences either through peer support or regular clinical supervision groups.
- Permission to attend the funerals of patients with whom they have worked closely, if the staff member wishes, as this can bring 'closure'.
- Ongoing education to raise awareness of self and others within a palliative care setting.
- Training that focuses not only on the care of dying patients but also on the impact this has on the caregivers.
- Managers can recognize the emotional demands placed upon staff and show them that they are valued.
- Acknowledgement that not all nurses are comfortable with or feel they have the necessary level of expertise to work in this field—with a regular review of developmental needs.
- Courses on stress management.
- Adequate staffing levels.

Some healthcare workers and relatives experience difficulty being in the presence of the dying, which means that, whilst the immediate physical needs of a patient are met, the emotional distress is neglected.

This distancing can often be attributed to not knowing what to say or how to act due to:

- discomfort at being put in touch with one's own mortality;
- not making time to become involved;
- feeling emotionally unable to contain the intensity of the situation;
- emotional distancing because dying is taking too long and is too painful to witness;
- anticipatory grief that can make it difficult to interact with the terminally ill patient;
- guilt and ambivalence experienced by those who feel they haven't been as supportive as they might have been;
- relief because suffering is coming to an end and guilt at feeling this.

Whereas CKD creates excessive pressure on families who are trying to integrate dialysis into their lives, terminal illness destroys future hopes and aspirations leaving families facing very different emotions. The prospect of dying is ever present and can reduce patients to waiting powerlessly for death. This is why we need to focus not so much on dying, but on helping patients identify and achieve what they want to accomplish whilst living. This requires recognition of the uniqueness of each individual patient, and working at their pace towards shared decision-making in terms of future treatment and end of life plans. The ability of staff to facilitate and manage cathartic interventions where patients can unburden themselves of fear and fantasies they hold around death and dying, can positively assist with their transition towards living whilst waiting to die.

Caring for the bereaved

Worden's identified tasks of mourning[1]

- Accepting the reality of loss
- Working through the pain and grief
- Adjusting to the loss
- Emotional relocation and acceptance

Both patients with CKD and their families have usually had a long association with their renal unit, and bereaved families often find enormous comfort remaining in touch with the hospital staff who have supported them over a great many years.

The difficulty some relatives experience in 'letting go' and moving on needs to be acknowledged and there are many ways in which the bereaved can be helped with this task. It is important that we do not let our own sense of helplessness keep us from reaching out to bereaved relatives and that we demonstrate genuine concern, care, and a willingness to listen and talk about the dead person.

Unlike hospices, for which bereavement support is an integral part of their service, renal units do not usually have the resources or expertise to provide bereavement care. However, support could be offered through:

- condolence cards or letters of sympathy;
- anniversary of death card for the first year;
- bereavement information leaflets that give not just practical help but also information on counselling availability in the locality or national organizations that offer this service;
- attending funerals;
- memorial services for those who have died within the past year.

Specialist palliative care services usually provide a bereavement service that is often targeted and might include:

- drop-in facilities;
- self-help groups;
- befriending schemes;
- professional or volunteer counselling;
- group therapy.

The availability of ongoing counselling for those who seek it has the potential to identify when the bereaved person is not progressing normally through their grief process and affords an opportunity for onward referral for more skilled help.

Support can also be obtained from the following.

- CRUSE (Tel : 0870 167 1677) www.crusebereavementcare.org.uk
- Compassionate Friends (Tel: 0845 1203785) www.tcf.org.uk

- National Bereavement Service: a 'support organization for the bereaved' that provides information on where they can access support locally; it also offers advice/counselling to people who ring their helpline (Tel: 020 7709 0505; Helpline Tel: 020 7709 9090).
- Bereavement—Patient UK www.patient.co.uk/showdoc
- Help for grieving children or their families www.winstonswish.org.uk

Reference

1 Worden JW (1991). *Grief counseling and grief therapy*. Springer, New York.

Drug doses in advanced chronic renal disease

Wendy Lawson

Drug handling in advanced chronic renal disease

Altered pharmacokinetics Numerous drugs are excreted by the kidney through glomerular filtration. When reduced this affects clearance of the drug and metabolites.

Absorption Absorption of drugs may be affected by excess urea generated by the internal urea ammonia cycle. This can result in gastric alkalization affecting absorption. Gastroparesis, nausea, vomiting, and anorexia may all reduce drug absorption.

Bioavailability This parameter varies more in patients with uraemia. Advanced uraemia alkalinizes saliva, which reduces bioavailability of drugs preferring an acid environment. Phosphate binders can form insoluble products with some drugs and decrease their absorption.

Volume of distribution (Vd) Following absorption, all drugs are distributed to different sites on the body depending on their volume of distribution. Vd represents the ratio of administered drug to the plasma concentration and indicates the degree of distribution or binding of a drug to tissues. It will be increased in patients with oedema or ascites for water-soluble drugs and decreased in muscle wasting or dehydration. Reduced doses are required to distribute into a smaller volume. Those patients with ascites or oedema may require higher drug doses. Drugs with a large Vd (e.g. > 0.6L/kg) are not confined within the circulation and tend to be lipid-soluble.

Protein binding The amount of 'free' drug or drug available to result in a desired therapeutic effect may depend on degree of protein binding, often to plasma albumin. Drugs that are highly protein bound, i.e. not available to exert a pharmacological effect, may compete with the retention of urea and other substances that compete for the plasma protein. Patients with CKD stage 5 frequently have reduced albumin levels and thus displaced drugs from binding, increasing plasma levels, pharmacological effect, and side-effects. Protein binding can also be altered by acid–base balance, malnutrition, and inflammation.

Drug metabolism The metabolism of drugs in the liver is affected by increased levels of urea. Drugs may be retained and exhibit pharmacological activity, e.g. morphine. Hydrolysis is often reduced; however, glucuronidation, microsomal oxidation, and sulphate conjugation can remain unchanged. Metabolism may be altered unpredictably in renal failure.

Renal excretion Excretion is often the main route of drug elimination. When reduced this affects active metabolites of some drugs, which are often eliminated renally. Toxic metabolites may accumulate.

Dosages of commonly used drugs in advanced chronic renal disease: introduction

Chronic kidney disease guidelines classify the condition into five stages (see Table 15.1). Stage 1 indicates normal or elevated glomerular filtration rate (GFR) with evidence of at least one parameter of chronic kidney damage while stage 5 (CKD5) indicates established renal failure where GFR < 15mL/min/1.73m^2.

GFR has been regularly estimated using the Cockcroft and Gault equation and subsequent drug dosage adjustments in renal impairment calculated. This uses body weight and takes extremities into account. More recently, another GFR prediction formula has been introduced and referred to as modification of diet in renal dosage (MDRD). The resultant estimated GFR (eGFR) does not require weight of patient and result is normalized to 1.73m^2.

Drug dosing in renal impairment published in the literature has been based on the Cockcroft and Gault calculation. This should be used unless references state that drug dosing has been expressed for normalizing eGFR.

The dosages outlined in Tables 15.2–15.8 represent those where GFR < 15mL/min and those used in clinical practice by authors of the text. The dosing guidelines are divided into CKD5 without or with support of haemodialysis.

Dosage guidance

Tables 15.2–15.8 list the dose adjustments for commonly used drugs in patients with CKD5. These patients may have withdrawn from dialysis support or may be in the latter stages of haemodialysis. Their creatinine clearance is < 15mL/min/1.73m^2. Published data may conflict on the specific doses to be used in this patient population. The tables provide data that take into consideration doses used in practice by clinicians who have provided data for this textbook. Where there is more than one formulation for a specific drug the form referred to is listed. If the dose and/or dosing interval have to be altered this is stated. Standard dose refers to dosage used in patients with normal renal function.

All doses should be confirmed with drug manufacturer's recommendations prior to use

Table 15.1 Classification of chronic kidney disease*

Stage	Description†	GFR (mL/min/1.73m²)
—	At increased risk for CKD	> 60 (with risk factors for CKD)
1	Kidney damage with normal GFR	≥ 90
2	Kidney damage with mildly decreased GFR	60–89
3	Moderately decreased GFR	30–59
4	Severely decreased GFR	15–29
5	Kidney failure	< 15 (or dialysis)

* Chronic kidney disease is defined as either kidney damage or a GFR < 60mL/min/1.73m² for 3 months or more.
† Kidney damage is defined as pathological abnormalities or markers of damage, including abnormalities in blood or urine tests or imaging studies.

Abbreviations used in Tables 15.2–15.8

—	unknown or no data available
Ch	chapter
CKD	chronic kidney disease
g	gram
HD	haemodialysis
IM	intramuscular
IV	intravenous
LD	loading dose
mcg	microgram
mg	milligram
on	every night
PO	oral
PR	rectally
prn	when required
q4h	every 4 hours
q6h	every 6 hours
q8h	every 8 hours
q24h	every 24 hours, etc.
SC	subcutaneous
SD	syringe driver
SL	sublingual

Drug dosages in CKD5: analgesics

See also 'Drugs to be avoided' and 'Drugs that do not need dosage modification' in CKD5 with or without dialysis (pp. 292 and 294) and additional notes on analgesics on p. 296.

Table 15.2 Analgesic drug dosing in CKD5 with and without haemodialysis

Drug	Serum half-life normal/ESRD (h)	% protein bound in normal renal function	Dosage for CKD5	
			Not on dialysis	With HD
Alfentanil	1–4/unchanged	88–95	For procedural or breakthrough pain: 200mcg SC or buccal/nasal spray (see Ch. 6). SD dose depends on previous opioid dose (see Chs. 6 & 12)	As for 'not on dialysis'
Buprenorphine	2.5–3/—	~96	See Ch. 6	As for 'not on dialysis'
Clonazepam	18–45/—	47–86	SC or PO: 0.5–2mg/24h (see Ch. 12)	As for 'not on dialysis'
Codeine phosphate	2.5–3.5/—	7	50% of standard dose	As for 'not on dialysis'
Fentanyl SC	2–7/unchanged	79–87	Depends on pain & previous opioid dose. Suggested starting dose opioid-naive: SD 100–200mcg/24h and titrate; bolus acute pain 12.5–25mcg (see Chs 6 & 12)	As for 'not on dialysis'
Fentanyl transdermal	17/unchanged	79–87	Established regime (see Chs 6 & 12)	As for 'not on dialysis'

Gabapentin	5–7/prolonged	< 3	300mg as single dose on alternative days	LD: for initial users 300–400mg. Maintenance: 200–300mg after HD on dialysis days only
Hydromorphone (non-modified release)	2.5/—	7.1	1.3mg q6h (see Ch. 6)	1.3mg 4–6h and titrate to response (see Ch. 6). Monitor carefully
Ibuprofen	2–3.2/unchanged	90–99	Avoid	Standard dose
Methadone	13–58/—	60–90	See Ch. 6	As for 'not on dialysis'
Oxycodone PO (non-modified release)	2/3–4	38	Limited evidence	Limited evidence Monitor carefully and see pp. 98–9
Paracetamol PO	2/unchanged	20–30	Standard dose or q6–8h	As for 'not on dialysis'
Pregabalin	—	—	Commence 25mg q24h & titrate to response	As for 'not on dialysis' but give dose after HD
Tramadol PO/IV (non-modified release)	6/11	4	50mg q12h	50mg q6h

Drug dosages in advanced CKD: antibiotics

See also 'Drugs to be avoided' and 'Drugs that do not need dosage modification' in CKD5 with or without dialysis (pp. 292 and 294).

Table 15.3 Antibiotic drug dosing in CKD5 with and without haemodialysis

Drug	Serum half-life normal/ESRD (h)	% protein bound in normal renal function	Dosage for CKD5	
			Not on dialysis	With HD
Amoxicillin IV/PO	0.9–2.3/5–20	15–25	Maximum 500mg q8h	As for 'not on dialysis'
Amoxicillin/ clavulanic acid IV/PO	Amoxicillin 0.9–2.3/ 5–20; clavulanic acid 1/3–4	15–25/30	Maximum PO 375mg q12h; IV 1.2g stat, then 600mg q24h	As for 'not on dialysis' but supplement IV 600mg post-HD
Benzylpenicillin	0.5/6–20	50	20–50% standard dose; maximum 3.6g/24h	As for 'not on dialysis'
Cefalexin	0.7/16	20	250–500mg q12h	As for 'not on dialysis'
Cefotaxime	1/15	13–37	1g LD; then 50% standard dose	50% standard dose
Ceftazidime	1.2/13–25	17	0.5–1g q24h	0.5–1g q24–48h
Cefuroxime IV	1.2/17	33	750mg–1.5g q12h	750mg–1.5g q24h
Ciprofloxacin IV/PO	3–6/6–9	20–40	50% standard dose	As for 'not on dialysis'

Clarithromycin IV/PO	2.3–6.0/6–9	50% standard dose	As for 'not on dialysis'
Erythromycin IV/PO	1.4/5–6	50–75% standard dose; max 1.5g/24h	As for 'not on dialysis'
Flucloxacillin IV/PO	0.8–1/3	Max PO 500mg q6h; IV up to 1g q6h	As for 'not on dialysis'
Metronidazole IV/PO	6–14/7–21	Standard dose q 12h	Standard dose
Piperacillin/tazobactam	Piperacillin 0.18–0.3/ 3.3–5.1; tazobactam 1/7	4.5g q12h	As for 'not on dialysis' but supplement 2.25g post-HD
Teicoplanin IV/IM	33–190/62–230	Days 1–3 standard dose; then day 4 standard dose q72h or 33% standard dose q24h	As for 'not on dialysis'
Trimethoprim PO	9–13/20–49	50% standard dose q24h	As for 'not on dialysis' but dose post-HD
Vancomycin IV	6–8/200–250	Stat dose & titrate to levels	As for 'not on dialysis'

Drug dosages in CKD5: antidepressants/antiemetics/antihistamines

See also 'Drugs to be avoided' and 'Drugs that do not need dosage modification' in CKD5 with or without dialysis (pp. 292 and 294).

Table 15.4 Antidepressant drug dosing in CKD5 with and without haemodialysis

Drug	Serum half-life normal/ESRD (h)	% protein bound in normal renal function	Dosage for CKD5	
			Not on dialysis	With HD
Dothiepin	14–24/—	80–90	Commence 25mg on & titrate to response	As for 'not on dialysis'
Fluoxetine	24–72h/4–6days (chronic dosing)	94.5	Standard dose or standard dose q48h	As for 'not on dialysis'
Nortriptyline	25–60/66–200	95	Reduce dose & titrate to response	As for 'not on dialysis'
Paroxetine	24/30	95	50% standard dose	As for 'not on dialysis'
Venlafaxine (non-modified release)	3.8/10.6	27	50% standard dose q24h	As for 'not on dialysis'

Table 15.5 Antiemetic/antihistamine drug dosing in CKD5 with and without haemodialysis

Drug	Serum half-life normal/ESRD (h)	% protein bound in normal renal function	Dosage for CKD5	
			Not on dialysis	With HD
Chlorpheniramine PO	14–24/—	72	4mg q6–8h	As for 'not on dialysis'
Domperidone	7.5/—	< 90	PO: 10–20mg q8h; PR: 30mg q12h	As for 'not on dialysis'
Haloperidol	10–40/—	90–92	PO or SC: 0.5–1.5mg q8h; SD: 1–3mg/24h	As for 'not on dialysis'
Levomepromazine	—	—	PO: 6mg or SC: 5mg up to q8h (see Ch. 12)	As for 'not on dialysis'
Metoclopramide IV/PM/PO	2.5–5.4/14–15	40	50% standard dose	As for 'not on dialysis'
Prochlorperazine	3–13/—	96	Reduce dose PO: 5mg; IM: 6.25mg & titrate to response	As for 'not on dialysis'

Drug dosages in CKD5: antipsychotic and antisecretory drugs

See also 'Drugs to be avoided' and 'Drugs that do not need dosage modification' in CKD5 with or without dialysis (pp. 292 and 294).

Table 15.6 Antipsychotic drug dosing in CKD5 with and without haemodialysis

Drug	Serum half-life normal/ESRD (h)	% protein bound in normal renal function	Dosage for CKD5	
			Not on dialysis	With HD
Chlorpromazine	11–42/unchanged	91–99	Reduce dose & titrate to response	As for 'not on dialysis'
Haloperidol	10–40/—	90–92	PO or SC: 0.5–1.5mg q8–24h	As for 'not on dialysis'
Olanzapine	30–38/37	93	5mg; then titrate	As for 'not on dialysis'
Pimozide	55–150/—	99	50% standard dose	As for 'not on dialysis'
Quetiapine	6–7/unchanged	83	25mg q24h, increasing in increments of 25–50mg q24h according to response	As for 'not on dialysis'
Risperidone	24/increased	88	PO: 0.5mg q12h, increasing by 0.5mg q12h to 1–2mg q12h	As for 'not on dialysis'
Trifluoperazine	7–18/—	< 99	50% standard dose if elderly/frail	As for 'not on dialysis'

Table 15.7 Antisecretory drug dosing in CKD5 with and without haemodialysis

Drug	Serum half-life normal/ESRD (h)	% protein bound in normal renal function	Dosage for CKD5	
			Not on dialysis	With HD
Glycopyrrolium*	1.7/—	—	SC: 200mcg stat & q4h prn SD: 600–1200mcg/24h	As for 'not on dialysis'
Hyoscine butylbromide	5–6/—	3–11	SC: 20mg stat & q2h prn SD: 40–160mg/24h (see Ch. 12)	As for 'not on dialysis'
Hyoscine hydrobromide	5–6/—	—	SC: 400mcg stat & q4h prn SD: 600–2400mcg/24h (see Ch. 12)	As for 'not on dialysis'
Ranitidine	2–3/6–9	15	50–100% standard dose	As for 'not on dialysis'

* Excreted by kidney so drug accumulates.

Notes on antipsychotics

• Psychotropic medications are highly protein bound in renal failure. This may mean that increased unbound/free drug is available to exert not only the desired therapeutic effect but also undesirable side-effects.

• Many of these medications require dosage titration according to response.

Drug dosages in CKD5: anxiolytics/hypnotics

See also 'Drugs to be avoided' and 'Drugs that do not need dosage modification' in CKD5 with or without dialysis (pp. 292 and 294).

Table 15.8 Anxiolytic/hypnotic drug dosing in CKD5 with and without haemodialysis

Drug	Serum half-life normal/ESRD (h)	% protein bound in normal renal function	Dosage for CKD5	
			Not on dialysis	With HD
Diazepam all forms	20–90/unchanged	94–99	Reduce dose; then titrate to response	As for 'not on dialysis'
Lorazepam all forms	5–10/32–70	85	Standard dose; titrate to response	As for 'not on dialysis'
Midazolam*	1.2–12.3/ unchanged	94–98	SC: 2.5mg q2h or SD: 10–20mg/24h (see Ch. 12)	As for 'not on dialysis'
Nitrazepam	18–50/unchanged	85	Reduce dose; then titrate to response	As for 'not on dialysis'
Oxazepam	6–25/25–90	97	10–20mg q6–8h	As for 'not on dialysis'
Temazepam	2–4/unchanged	96–98	Reduce dose & titrate up to 10mg on (20mg if single dose)	As for 'not on dialysis'
Zopiclone	3.5–6/77	45–80	3.75–7.5mg on	As for 'not on dialysis'

Notes on anxiolytics

* Active metabolites accumulate in renal failure.
+ Parent drug can accumulate in renal failure.
• Diazepam. Commence with reduced dosage and titrate to response.
• Oxazepam. There is an increase in volume of distribution and reduction in protein binding; therefore decrease dose.

Some drugs not requiring dosage alteration in CKD5 with or without haemodialysis

Amitriptyline
Bisacodyl
Carbamazepine
Cefuroxime (oral)
Clopidogrel
Cyclizine
Dexamethasone
Domperidone
Doxepin
Enoxaparin (prophylaxis dose)
Esomeprazole
Granisetron
Heparin (unfractionated)
Imipramine
Isosorbide mono/dinitrate
Lactulose
Lansoprazole
Levothyroxine
Nystatin suspension
Octreotide
Omeprazole
Ondansetron
Pantoprazole
Paracetamol
Phenoxymethylpenicillin
Phenytoin
Remifentanyl
Senna
Sertraline
Sevelamer
Sodium valproate
Terfenadine
Triazolam
Trifluoperazine
Tropisetron
Zolpidem

Some drugs to avoid in CKD5 with or without haemodialysis

ACE inhibitors
Aluminium- and magnesium-containing antacids
Angiotensin-11 receptor antagonists
Aminoglycosides
Aspirin (therapeutic doses)
Cyclo-oxygenase 2 inhibitors
Dextropropoxyphene
Dihydrocodeine
Enoxaparin (therapeutic dose)
Gaviscon®
Glibenclamide
Gliclazide
Glipizide
Lofepramine
Mefazodone
Metformin
Morphine
Nitrofurantoin
NSAIDs (unless on HD)
Peptac®
Pethidine
Thiazides
Thioridazine

Notes on analgesics and further reading

Notes on analgesics (see Chapter 6)

- Choice of analgesics may depend on a number of factors including cause of pain (which is often multifactorial), effect of current treatment regimen, and severity of pain.
- The principles of the World Health Organization (WHO) three-step analgesic ladder can be applied to the management of pain in patients with CKD stage 5, both those on and not on haemodialysis, though there are minor differences in doses highlighted in Chapter 6 and the Table 15.2. The commonest reason for modifying analgesic dose is that toxicity can occur due to accumulation of active metabolites. All analgesics require individual monitoring and dosage titration.
- See Chapter 6 for full discussion of individual strong opioids.
- Sustained release forms of opioids should not be used as if accumulation occurs there may be prolonged toxicity.
- Subcutaneous drivers–it is important to check compatibility with other drugs.

Further reading

Ashley C, Currie A (2004). *The renal drug handbook*, 2nd edn. Radcliffe Press, Oxford.

Cohen LM, Tessier EG, Germain MJ, *et al.* (2004). Update on psychotropic medications use in renal disease. *Psychosomatics* **45**, 34–48.

Devaney A, Ashley C, Tomson C (2006). How the reclassification of kidney disease impacts on dosing adjustments. *Pharm J* **277**, 403–4.

Dickman A, Schneider J, Varga J (2005). *The syringe driver: continuous subcutaneous infusions in palliative care*. Oxford University Press, Oxford.

Electronic Medicines Compendium *www. medicines.org.uk* Accessed December 2006.

Murtagh FEM, Addington-Hall JM, Donohoe P, *et al.* (2006). Symptom management in patients with established renal failure: management without dialysis. *EDTA/ERCA J* **32** (2), 93–8.

Ferro CJ, Chambers EJ, Davison SN (2004). Management of pain in renal failure. In *Supportive care for the renal patient* (ed. EJ Chambers, M Germain, E Brown), pp. 105–53. Oxford University Press, Oxford.

Germain M, McCarthy S (2004). Symptoms of renal disease: dialysis related symptoms. In *Supportive care for the renal patient* (ed. EJ Chambers, M Germain, E Brown), pp. 75–94. Oxford University Press, Oxford.

Useful website *www.palliativedrugs.com*

Resources

Patients and carers

The most commonly expressed concerns that renal patients or their families raise when terminal or end of life issues are discussed relate to the level of financial help and practical help they can expect to receive.

Benefits The main benefits are the following.

Disability Living Allowance (DLA)/Attendance Allowance (AA) The legal definition of terminal illness under Section 66(2)() of the Social Security Contributions and Benefit Act 1992 provides that you count as being terminally ill at any time 'if at that time (you have) a progressive disease and (your) death in consequence of that disease can reasonably be expected within 6 months'.

Such patients can claim the Disability Living Allowance or Attendance Allowance under special rules that require a doctor's DS1500 report to be completed and forwarded with the application. This will enable the 3-month qualifying period to be waived allowing patients to immediately receive the highest weekly rate of benefit for help with personal care and for mobility if the criteria are met.

Blue badges can also be awarded to people who are in receipt of the higher rate mobility component of the DLA, are blind, or 'have a permanent and substantial disability which causes inability to walk or very considerable difficulty in walking'. Applications should be made to the Concessionary Fares Department of the patient's local authority.

Carer's allowance Claimants need to be over 16 and spending at least 35 hours a week caring for a person who is in receipt of the AA or DLA (at the middle or highest rate for personal care). You are not eligible to claim if you are in full time education with 21 hours or more a week of supervised study or earn more than £84 per week after certain deductions.

Further information on benefit eligibility

Citizens Advice Bureau www.citizensadvice.org.uk
Benefit Enquiry Line: free phone 0800 882200
National Kidney Federation Helpline: Tel 0845 6010209
www.kidney.org.uk email helpline@kidney.org.uk
www.direct.gov.uk
Counsel and Care. Advice line 0845 300 7585 offers advice on community care, benefits, care at home, residential care, and financial help for older people.

Practical help

- Disability Discrimination Act (1995) defines disability as 'physical or mental impairment which has a substantial and long-term adverse effect on (your) ability to carry out normal day to day activities'. Further information from the Disability Rights Commission Helpline 0845 762 2633 or www.drc-gb.org
- Community care. The first step towards obtaining community care services is an assessment of needs. Social services currently has the lead role but local authorities have a duty to invite the NHS to assist if there is a health need and they are required to work closely together using pooled budgets and joint commissioning of services

to provide the most appropriate level of care for the patient (NHS and Community Care Act 1990).
- Carers are also entitled to an assessment of need in their own right (Carers (Recognition and Services) Act 1995).

Support for carers

- Carers UK (Tel 020 7490 8818; free phone Carers' Line 0808 808 7777) provides information and advice on all aspects of caring to both carers and professionals.
- Crossroads—Caring for Carers (Tel 0845 450 0350) is committed to providing practical support where it is most needed. Trained carer support workers take over caring tasks in the home to provide carers with a break www.crossroads.org.uk
- Princess Royal Trust (Tel 020 7480 7788) provides free and confidential help for all carers.
- Department of Health caring about Carers: Carers UK www.carers.gov.uk
- Expert Patient Programme—'Looking after me' provides training in self-managing the stresses and emotions that arise as a result of being a carer www.expertpatients.co.uk
- British Kidney Patients Association (Tel 014200 472021) offers financial help and advice to patients and carers.

Useful websites

www.carersonline.org.uk
www.dss.gov.uk
www.disabilityalliance.org

After a death

Following a death there can be many practical issues to deal with.
- If a death occurs in hospital or in a hospice, the ward staff should have leaflets, such as DWP D49 'What to do after a death in England and Wales' or D49S 'What to do after a death in Scotland',that give advice and information about all aspects of bereavement.
- If a death occurs at home, the district nurse should be able to offer advice.
- Practical help and advice is also available from funeral directors, GPs, solicitors, religious organizations, social service departments, and the Citizens' Advice Bureau.

Organizations offering support

Age Concern is an organization that can offer pre- and post-death advice and support. Tel 020 8765 7200; information line 0800 009966; http://www.ageconcern.org.uk

Cruse Bereavement Care (Tel 0870 167 1677) provides bereavement support, information, advice, and support groups. http://www.crusebereavementcare.org.uk

Compassionate Friends (Tel 0845 120 3785; Helpline 0845 1232304) offers nationwide support from bereaved parent to bereaved parent and their immediate families. http://www.tcf.org.uk

Winston's Wish (Tel 0845 2030405) offers a service to bereaved families and young people. http://www.winstonswish.org.uk

Bereavement—patient UK. www.patient.co.uk/showdoc

Professionals

Palliative medicine

Drug information

- This site provides essential, comprehensive, and independent information for health professionals about the use of drugs in palliative care. It highlights drugs given for unlicensed indications or by unlicensed routes and the administration of multiple drugs by continuous SC infusion *http://www.palliativedrugs.com*
- The Cochrane Pain, Palliative, and Supportive Care Group (PaPaS) focuses on reviews for the prevention and treatment of pain; the treatment of symptoms at the end of life; and supporting patients, carers, and their families through the disease process. *http://www.jr2.ox.ac.uk/cochrane*

Community palliative care The Gold Standards Framework (GSF) is a systematic approach to optimizing the care delivered by primary care teams for any patient nearing the end of life in the community. *http://www.goldstandardsframework.nhs.uk/non_cancer.php*

End of life care

- The Liverpool Care Pathway for the dying patient (LCP) has been developed to transfer the hospice model of care into other care settings. *http://www.lcp-mariecurie.org.uk*
- The Preferred Place of Care Plan (PPC) is intended to be a patient-held record that will follow the patient through their path of care into the variety of differing health and social care settings. *http://www.cancerlancashire.org.uk/ppc.html*
- **Organizations** The National Council for Palliative Care (NCPC) is the umbrella organization for all those who are involved in providing, commissioning, and using palliative care and hospice services in England, Wales, and Northern Ireland. NCPC promotes the extension and improvement of palliative care services for all people with life-threatening and life-limiting conditions. NCPC promotes palliative care in health and social care settings across all sectors to government, national, and local policy-makers. *http://www.ncpc.org.uk*

Renal medicine

- The UK Renal Registry provides annual reports about treatment of end-stage renal disease in the UK. *http://www.renalreg.com*
- The Renal Association is the professional association for renal physicians. Provides links to most renal websites in UK, documents about providing renal care, information about renal courses in UK. *http://www.renal.org*
- Renal NSF Part 2 provides guidelines of good practice for end of life management and patient choice in renal disease. *http://www.dh.gov.uk/PublicationsAndStatistics/Publications/PublicationsPolicyAndGuidance/Browsable/DH_4102941*

Index

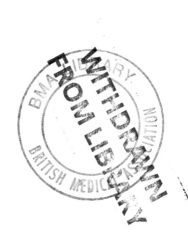